THE
RETINOSCOPY
BOOK

**An Introductory Manual
for Eye Care Professionals**

Fifth Edition

THE RETINOSCOPY BOOK

An Introductory Manual for Eye Care Professionals

Fifth Edition

John M. Corboy, MD

Former Associate Clinical Professor of Surgery (Ophthalmology)
John A. Burns School of Medicine
University of Hawaii
Honolulu, Hawaii

Former Faculty Joint Commission on Allied Health
Personnel in Ophthalmology

With:
David Norath, COT
Ron Stone, CRA
Richard Reffner, COT

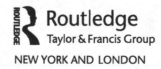

NEW YORK AND LONDON

Medical Illustrations by: Susie Young Anderson

First published in 2005 by SLACK Incorporated

Published 2024 by Routledge
605 Third Avenue, New York, NY 10017
4 Park Square, Milton Park, Abingdon, Oxon OX14 4RN

Routledge is an imprint of the Taylor & Francis Group, an informa business

Corboy, John M.
    The retinoscopy book : an introductory manual for eye care
professionals / John Corboy, with David Norath ... [et al.].-- 5th ed.
        p. ; cm.
    Includes bibliographical references and index.
    ISBN 1-55642-623-2 (pbk. : alk. paper)
    1. Retinoscopy--Handbooks, manuals, etc.
    [DNLM: 1. Refractive Errors--diagnosis. 2.
Optometry--instrumentation. 3. Optometry--methods. 4. Refraction,
Ocular. WW 300 C792r 2003] I. Title.
    RE928.C672 2003
    617.7'55--dc21

                                2003002379

ISBN: 9781556426230 (pbk)
ISBN: 9781003526322 (ebk)

DOI: 10.1201/9781003526322

DEDICATION

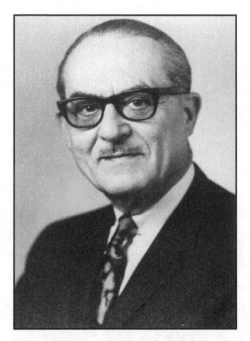

To the memory of Jack C. Copeland, the father of streak retinoscopy, who developed the retinoscope and spent his life teaching its use, this book is gratefully dedicated.

CONTENTS

PREFACE TO THE FIFTH EDITION

In the 24 years since this book was first published, I have been delighted with its continued success as a teaching device for ophthalmic technicians, ophthalmology residents, and optometrists.

While there have been improvements in autorefractors, in my offices there is just no substitute for mastery of these skills. We continue to value "retinoscopy techs" above all others, and to compensate them appropriately.

With the popularity of refractive surgery, the need has come to evaluate the sometimes peculiar reflexes seen postoperatively. Our chief tech, Ron Stone, CRA, has graciously provided a new chapter demonstrating this art, as well as a needed section on instrument maintenance.

In recent years, there has been a gradual increase in the number of practices using minus cylinder refractors, although I can't imagine why. Dave J. Norath, COT, has kindly amplified on minus cylinder techniques for this edition. Dave has also added a helpful chapter on concave mirror retinoscopy.

We have been impressed by the usefulness of methods for mounting the schematic eye on the headrest of the examination chair, thus using the lenses in the refractor to perform the retinoscopy exercises in this manual. This eliminates the need for a separate trial case of lenses and gives the technician a more "real life" experience from the beginning. My former chief ophthalmic technician, Rich Reffner, COT, has kindly written and illustrated the section showing how you can do this.

The marketplace in instruments has changed since the last edition. We are grateful to the manufacturers who have provided updated photos and pricing.

I want to thank Fran Schoen and the staff of the Joint Commission on Allied Health Personnel in Ophthalmology for their support with my retinoscopy and refractometry courses over the years and my publisher, SLACK Incorporated, for encouraging this new edition.

Finally, I want to thank hundreds of retinoscopy students over the decades who have told me of their pleasure and satisfaction with this manual. The process of writing is a great teacher, for by the time a book is finished the author has invariably learned far more than he knew to start with. Here's hoping this new edition proves even more valuable.

Mahalo nui loa,

John M. Corboy, MD
Kaunakakai, Molokai
2003

PREFACE TO THE FIRST EDITION

No technique in daily use by modern ophthalmic practitioners has received less written attention than retinoscopy. Refraction and optic texts say little about the subject, and many beginners rely on the instructions that accompany their first instrument. Most students take an introductory course of some kind, and after struggling through months or years of trial and error, develop a measure of confidence and skill.

Courses vary markedly in quality, for there are not many teachers of refraction—much less of retinoscopy—sufficiently available, interested, and capable of clearly presenting the fundamentals. The few instruction manuals, which are relatively intelligible to the experienced retinoscopist, often appear almost incomprehensible to the novice.

My attempt here is to put together a comprehensive introduction to the subject in a small package, so that even the solitary student, alone with the schematic eye and a trial case, can find his way. This book can in no way substitute for an inspired instructor, but in the absence of one, it should prove helpful.

My preoccupation with retinoscopy dates from 1966, when, as one of a group of first-year Washington University eye residents, I took a short course in the subject from its master, Jack Copeland. He knew all the intricacies, but many of us were scarcely able to understand the basics.

As a result, I set out to master the subject on my own by working late at night at the McMillan Library. There, with my schematic eye, I began to construct diagrams representing cones of emerging light, labeled WITH and AGAINST.

When later I was asked to teach retinoscopy, I tried to help my students escape my own early frustrations by setting out in a syllabus the method I had evolved for my own benefit.

It is my conviction that the retinoscope is second only to the slitlamp as the most useful instrument in ophthalmology. Despite the theoretical promise of automated refraction, skill in retinoscopy is essential, as is patience with its mastery. While none of us may prove as brilliant in its use as Jack Copeland,

we can acquire the fundamentals and then, with review of his advanced techniques, grasp the subtleties of objective refraction.

Explanations that rely heavily on vergence formulas and other unfamiliar optical principles usually discourage newcomers to retinoscopy. Yet the familiar cookbook approach ("if you see 'with motion,' add plus…") leaves many questions unanswered as well, and fails to build a framework of understanding.

The method I use attempts to demonstrate graphically why we see and do things, while avoiding the mathematics and ray diagrams that seem to confuse beginners. There is plenty of time to derive the formulas later, but in my courses, we have patients to refract by the 12th hour.

Admittedly, it is not easy to teach optical principles without a single equation or acknowledgment of Snell's law; this simplistic approach will be faulted by purists and criticized by the experienced, but perhaps it will continue to serve those beginners for whom it is intended.

Beginning retinoscopists arrive in various states of preparedness, but I have found it best to assume that most have a very limited knowledge of optics. In a classroom setting, a teacher tailors the presentation to the level of the audience; for this book, I am obligated to address the least sophisticated student, and consequently I amplify explanations and definitions. For more facile readers, this may involve some tiresome repetition.

In an art with many variations, I have stuck to what I know best, and to what seems to find general acceptance: streak retinoscopy with plus cylinders, using chiefly static methods. I hope the reader will realize that the introductory techniques taught here make a concession to brevity and simplicity, and that he will later seek to develop proficiency in more advanced methods, especially estimation techniques.

Use this book to teach yourself. From Chapter 5 on, you will need a schematic eye and trial lens case; most students buy the former and borrow the latter from their friendly local eye doc.

I would like to acknowledge those who have contributed to the production of this book; My mentors Jay Enoch, Ben Milder, and James Lebensohn taught me the fun and the challenge in "routine" refraction; Jay Enoch urged me to try teaching the unteachable; Jack Hartstein kept me at it; the ophthalmology residents who found this method useful encouraged me to put it between covers; and my artist, Susie Young Anderson, cheerfully hung in there through countless deadlines, turning my sketches into these excellent illustrations.

I owe much to Paul "Doc" Berry, my friend and editor, who likes to manipulate words; to Steve Michael, our patient photographer; to Corky Trinidad, cartoonist; and to Barney Copeland and Walter Gager, who provided perspective; to Dick Cole, Linda Burger, Arnold Stenner, Darv Guthmiller, Dion Bradshaw; Bruce Walters, Jerry Nelson, and other manufacturers' representatives, who gave valuable assistance; to Cecilia Tamondong, Pam Koerner Dooley and Mac McClain, who put up with the manuscript; and to Jackie Gould Fry, my office manager, who put up with me; to my wife Mary Jo, who gave me unfailing support; and to the many "friends of Bill Wilson and Doctor Bob," without whom nothing would have been accomplished.

I hope you enjoy learning from this book, and I welcome your suggestions for clarifying the next edition.

Aloha!

John M. Corboy, MD
Wahiawa, Hawaii
1979

FOREWORD

In an age of rapidly advancing computer technology in the ophthalmic sciences, it is refreshing to see a down-to-earth approach to an art that dates to the 19th century. John Corboy has written a practical treatise concerning a priceless part of the diagnostic armamentarium of all those who deal with physiologic optics. Retinoscopy (skiametry) is as valuable to the refractionist as a scalpel to a surgeon.

When the father of streak retinoscopy, Jack C. Copeland, introduced the first variable vergence streak retinoscope in the early 1920s, he accompanied it with a written monograph describing the instrument's use, thereby laying the foundation for basic streak retinoscopy. During the next 45 years, he traveled the world, teaching and honing his techniques. Copeland influenced generations of refractionists with a rapid, accurate, "new" method of objective refraction. Shortly before his death, Copeland developed a newer instrument designed to utilize all the detailed techniques he had observed and taught. Unfortunately, he did not leave a chronicle of his accomplishments, and his monograph was inadequate to teach the full scope of the instrument or to indicate the potential of retinoscopy.

The novice retinoscopist may fail to appreciate the importance of many subtle reflex nuances because of the absence of basic instruction in the use of the instrument, and also because of ignorance of the meaning of pupillary images produced by the instrument. In some cases, the basic techniques of retinoscopy are handed down from year to year by instructors who learned it wrong initially. In other cases, instructors did not take time to learn all the uses of this versatile instrument.

To become an accomplished retinoscopist, an intimate knowledge of physiologic and mathematical optics is not mandatory. What is imperative is initial training in correct use of the retinoscope, as well as an accurate knowledge of its capabilities. The practitioner who learns these basics, and then develops complete mastery of reflex interpretation through determined, thoughtful practice, can measure the refractive error in any individual with a high degree of accuracy and confidence. Dr. Corboy presents here this basic information and describes other advanced tools of skiametry in a comprehensive, readable, and inexpensive text. It is, in sum, a complete course in clinical retinoscopy.

Walter E. Gager, MD

RETINOSCOPY
ITS USE AND DEVELOPMENT

"You can't learn retinoscopy by reading a book…"

Jack C. Copeland

Retinoscopy is an objective method of measuring the optical power of the eye. We use a retinoscope to illuminate the inside of the eye and to observe the light that is reflected from the retina. These reflected rays change as they pass out through the optical components of the eye, and by examining just how these emerging rays change, we determine the refractive power of the eye.

We describe retinoscopy as *objective* because we evaluate the eye as an optical instrument, initially ignoring any information the eye transmits to the brain. Thus, retinoscopy does not depend on the patient's vision or judgment.

After we have objectively determined the refraction, we may then ask the patient to evaluate or *refine* our findings, a procedure that goes beyond what we specifically refer to as retinoscopy. If the patient approves of the correcting lens we have found via retinoscopy, he or she subjectively confirms our measurements. On the other hand, if the objective findings do not coincide with the subjective response, we can recheck both sources of information.

Retinoscopy reduces refraction time and error by quickly producing the approximate correcting lens, thereby minimizing the decisions the patient must make to refine the correction.

As an objective test, retinoscopy proves invaluable in situations where communication is difficult or impossible, such as with children or developmentally disabled persons. For the infant with poor vision and the foreigner who has lost his glasses, or for the deaf or senile patient, retinoscopy provides the *only* way to handle the problems of refraction.

By evaluating the retinoscopic reflex, we can also detect aberrations of the cornea and of the lens, as well as opacities of the ocular media.

RETINOSCOPY AS ART

Because we subjectively interpret the reflex in order to arrive at our objective measurements, retinoscopy qualifies as an art, and as with other arts, it proves rewarding to those willing to work through the initial difficulties. Skillful retinoscopy will save you many hours and much frustration in refraction, and it can be tremendously satisfying to you and your patients.

With practice, retinoscopy will provide you with exact measurement of refractive errors, but long before you develop skill in this technique, you will find retinoscopy a valuable starting point for every refraction. As each patient appraises the lens you have chosen for him or her, you will learn to improve your techniques, and in time, achieve a degree of real confidence in your measurements.

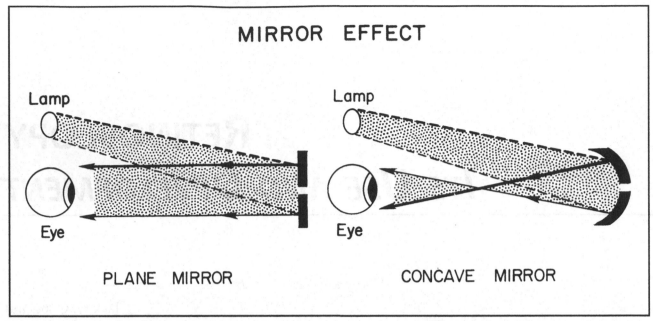

Figure 1-1. Mirror retinoscopy. The plane mirror emits essentially parallel, uncrossed rays. The concave mirror converges rays to a point from which they cross and diverge; this usually produces an opposite reflex or reversed motion.

It is difficult to imagine relying on trial and error methods rather than on retinoscopy, yet this invaluable diagnostic tool has evolved only recently.

EVOLUTION OF RETINOSCOPY

The story of the discovery and development of retinoscopy is an absorbing tale of observation, diligence, and good fortune. The everyday techniques that we take for granted come from many contributions by pioneers in physiologic optics. If you are interested, I recommend Millodot's brief historical review, which contains a good bibliography.[1]

In 1859, Sir William Bowman commented on the peculiar linear fundus reflex he saw when viewing astigmatic eyes with Helmholtz's new ophthalmoscope. Until Bowman described a technique for detecting astigmatism in keratoconus, refractive errors were assessed by purely subjective methods.

The first objective diagnosis of refractive errors was by the French ophthalmologist Cuignet in 1873, using a simple mirror ophthalmoscope (which reflected lamplight into the eye). Through the peephole in his mirror, Cuignet observed a curious reflex that varied among persons with differing refractive errors (Figure 1-1).

Cuignet discovered that when light from the *plane* mirror was moved across the pupil, the reflection from the fundus moved also; sometimes in the same direction, but often in the reverse direction. The speed of the movement, as well as the size and brightness of the reflex, varied among individuals. Sometimes the direction of movement varied in different meridians; that is, if Cuignet moved the light horizontally, the reflex might move in the same direction, while if he moved the light vertically, the reflex might travel in a reverse direction.

Cuignet attributed the reflexes he saw to the cornea and called his technique *keratoscopie.* In spite of his error, he was able with his mirror to *qualitatively* assess refractive errors, classifying them as myopia, hyperopia, or astigmatism. So we honor Cuignet as the father of retinoscopy.

As is often the case, it took a disciple to work out the doctrinal flaws and spread the message. Mengin, an often overlooked student of Cuignet, accepted Landolt's suggestion that the fundus was the actual source of the reflexes. In 1878, Mengin published the clear and simple explanation that helped to popularize this novel technique.

Meanwhile, another Frenchman, Parent, had worked out the optics to the point where he could actually measure the refractive error with lenses. In

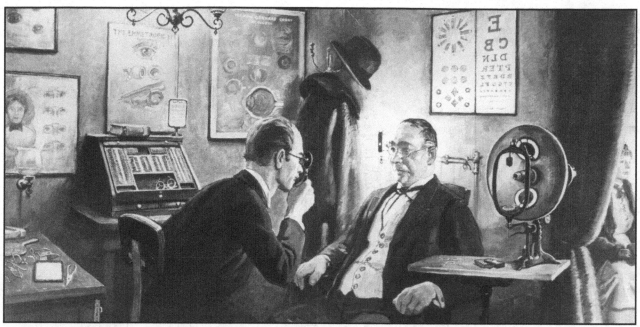

Figure 1-2. Retinoscopy at the turn of the century. The refractionist is using a mirror retinoscope to reflect rays from the gaslight into the eye, while studying the fundus reflex through the peephole (photo courtesy of American Optical Co).

1880, he published his explanation of quantified objective refraction. To emphasize the role of the retina, Parent proposed the term *retinoscopie*, but later, at the suggestion of a linguist, chose the term *skiascopie* (skia meaning shadow). Many other terms were proposed but abandoned; they included dioptroscopy, pupilloscopy (korescopy), umbrascopy, and scotoscopy.

The term *retinoscopy* is usually used in English, but it is imprecise because the retina is transparent and is not actually the source of reflexes seen with the retinoscope. Nevertheless, after a century of use the term carries a meaning of its own. The more correct word, *skiascopy*, is used throughout the rest of the world, and occasionally, you will see the instrument referred to as a *retinascope*.

NEW THEORIES INTRODUCED

Further explanations and theories were offered by Priestly-Smith, Donders, Gullstrand, Wolff, and others. In 1903, Duane first advocated the systematic use of *cylindrical* lenses for retinoscopy in astigmatism. Purists have often enjoyed debating the finer points of theoretical optics to explain just how retinoscopy really works. Landolt's *far point* theory,

which forms the basis for most of our present understanding, has been challenged by the observer-pupil theory of Wolff and the photokinetic theory of Haass.[2]

The gaslight (Figure 1-2) was later replaced by an incandescent lamp. Before long, a miniature bulb was developed that could be placed within the instrument, thus producing the *luminous* retinoscope. These electrified marvels projected a spot of light, much like a modern ophthalmoscope. Later designs with *variable vergence* produced plane and concave mirror effects from the same instrument.

Spot retinoscopes have not changed much in 100 years. Despite their limitations, these instruments remain in use today. Occasionally, you will be advised to choose a spot retinoscope for learning fundamentals, advancing to a streak model only when you have mastered certain techniques. This can be likened to a beginning driver training in a Model T. Streak retinoscopy is more accurate, and it is actually simpler and faster—even for a novice.

About the time reflecting retinoscopes were being replaced by the luminous models, other instruments and techniques began evolving. From the beginning, the founders of ophthalmic optics had appreciated the *linear* fundus reflex seen in

Figure 1-3. The original Copeland streak retinoscope.

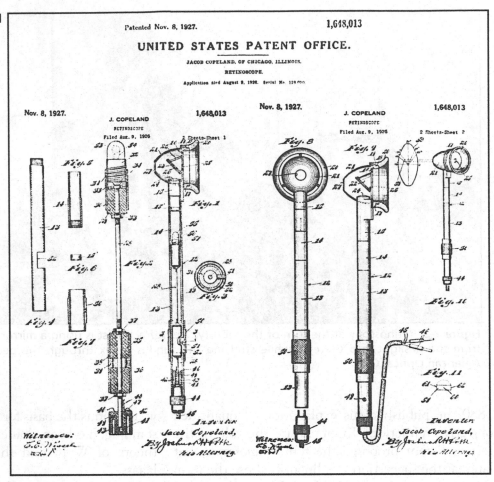

astigmatism. Around the turn of the century, Jackson, Wolff, and others emphasized the value of enhancing this reflex. With various slit-shaped mirrors they created a linear beam (or streak) of light, and the streak retinoscope was born. The streak reflex simplified refraction in astigmatism; later, an electric retinoscope with a rotating slit was devised to allow easier comparison of the ocular meridians.

COPELAND'S CONTRIBUTIONS

Around 1920, a serendipitous event occurred that changed the course of retinoscopy. A young optical genius named Jack C. Copeland was studying astigmatic reflexes:

"Jack was using one of Wolff's original European spot retinoscopes, when he dropped the instrument on the floor, damaging the bulb filament. When reexamining the schematic eye that he was working with, he noted a difference in the reflexes, and set about solving what had happened. From this original observation came the streak retinoscopic technique that is taught today."
—Walter E. Gager, MD (personal correspondence)

From his study of the linear reflex produced by the bent filament, Copeland devised an ingenious bulb that projected a linear beam of light. He then designed an instrument that rotated the bulb, so he could turn the streak through all the ocular meridians. The Copeland streak retinoscope also incorporated variable vergence and an improved mirror with a vertically oval pupil (to correct aberrations in the reflex). His original model, patented in 1927, popularized the streak technique and revolutionized retinoscopy (Figure 1-3).

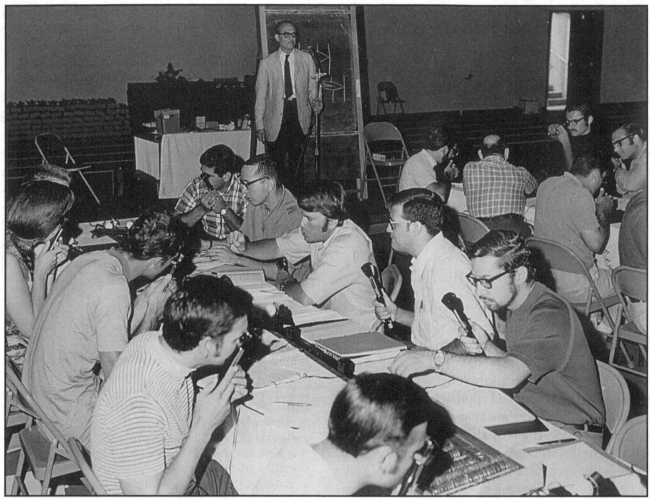

Figure 1-4. Jack Copeland, shortly before his death, doing what he did best: teaching retinoscopy (photo courtesy of Walter E. Gager, MD).

While most of the elements of Copeland's instrument had historical precedent, his invention incorporated all the important components into one unique design, one that was not improved upon for 40 years, and then by Copeland himself.

The streak retinoscope allows refraction of individual ocular meridians and rapid comparison of the principal meridians. With the streak we can accurately determine the astigmatic axis and the power of the correcting cylinder. Most of the retinoscopes sold in United States in the past 60 years have been streak models.

Copeland not only provided the instrument, but developed and popularized an entire system of objective refraction. Streak retinoscopy, as taught by Copeland, is *plus cylinder* retinoscopy; astigmatism is measured and corrected by convex (plus)

cylinders. By modifying this technique, as we shall see later, we can adapt streak retinoscopy to minus cylinders (see Chapter 10).

The most venerable retinoscope in the United States is the original Copeland design manufactured (with only minor changes) by Bausch & Lomb for 70 years. This instrument has five flaws that Copeland corrected in his improved version, marketed since 1968 as the Optec 360 (Stereo Optical Co, Chicago, Ill) (see Chapter 2, Figure 2-1). Several manufacturers have modified the original design, and each instrument has certain advantages. The various retinoscopes are described in the next chapter.

For more than 45 years, until his death in 1973, Copeland conducted thousands of courses and seminars as the foremost retinoscopy instructor in the country (Figure 1-4). The fundamentals of his technique are contained in the instruction booklets that accompany the Copeland instruments. They were also published as a chapter in Sloane's manual.[3]

Considering the time an ophthalmic practitioner spends daily with his or her retinoscope, surprisingly little of substance has been written about the technique. Copeland's descriptions of his method, while comprehensible to the experienced retinoscopist, have always somewhat baffled neophytes. The beginner, with little grasp of basic optics, has difficulty learning retinoscopy. The instrument is foreign, the terms new, judgments subjective, and the images but fleeting shadows.

OTHER CONTRIBUTIONS

Weinstock and Wirtschafter analyzed Copeland's writings, organized his method, and presented a decision-oriented, step-by-step approach to retinoscopy.[4] Their method has been expanded into a book that will appeal to those who prefer a highly structured, programmed approach.[5]

Automated refractors are now available that perform retinoscopy, compute the refraction, and print out the result through the use of infrared light. Their bulk, cost, and temperamental nature have all been reduced, making them increasingly popular. Electronic machines can do the job much faster. When retinoscopy is useless (eg, in opacities of the media or corneal irregularities) so are these devices. Nevertheless, they speed up part of the examination in many patients.[6]

Please bear in mind, however, that retinoscopy alone (whether by man or machine) does not produce a prescription for lenses; it does not tell you what the patient sees, or even *if* he or she sees. As an objective evaluation of the refractive state, retinoscopy is subject to specific, predictable errors. A proper *refraction* consists of objective *measurements* combined with a subjective *refinement* of these by the patient. Since an experienced retinoscopist usually spends only a minute on retinoscopy and a much longer time on subjective refinement, electronic devices do not save much time with most patients. Until automated refractors are as portable, inexpensive, and trouble-free as a retinoscope, there will remain a need for skilled retinoscopists. In my office, I've tried most models and find them disappointing; I much prefer a good retinoscopist.

REFERENCES

1. Millodot M. A centerary of retinoscopy. *J Am Optometric Assoc.* 1973;44:1057-1059.

2. Kettesy A. Uber die theorein der skiaskopic anlasslich ihress 100 jahrigen bestehens. *Klinische Monatsblauer fur Augenheilkunde.* 1973;162:26-33.

3. Copeland JC. Streak Retinoscopy. In: Sloane AE, ed. *Manual of Refraction.* 2nd ed. Boston, Mass: Little, Brown, and Co; 1970:83,102,106.

4. Weinstock SM, Wirtschafter JD. A decision-oriented flow chart for teaching and performing retinoscopy. *Trans Am Acad Ophthalmol Otolaryngol.* 1973;77:732-738.

5. Weinstock SM, Wirtschafter JD. *A Decision-oriented Manual of Retinoscopy.* Springfield, Ill: Charles C. Thomas; 1976:6,99.

6. Rubin ML, Volk D, Saffir A, et al. Symposium automatic refractions. *Trans Am Acad Ophthalmol and Otolaryngol.* 1975;79:481-512S.

THE RETINOSCOPE
HOW IT WORKS

"There's less in a retinoscope than meets the eye..."

Paul ("Doc") Berry

The majority of retinoscopes in use today employ the streak projection system developed by Copeland. For simplicity, we will confine this discussion to popular streak retinoscopes.

The exterior common to all streak retinoscopes appears in Figure 2-1. You look through the peephole along the beam projected out the opposite side of the *head*. Raising or lowering the *sleeve* changes the focus (vergence) of the beam, while turning the sleeve rotates the projected streak. The *handle* provides the power source.

Now let's examine what happens inside. The design and use of the instrument become clear when you see them as separate systems: one for projection and the other for observation.

PROJECTION SYSTEM

The projection system illuminates the retina and contains these major components:

- **Light source**: A bulb with a linear filament that projects a line or streak of light. Turning the sleeve on the instrument rotates the bulb, which, in turn, rotates the projected streak. This turning sleeve and the rotating of the light streak we call *meridian control* (Figure 2-2).

- **Condensing lens**: Resting in the light path, the lens focuses rays from the bulb onto the mirror (Figure 2-3).

- **Mirror**: Placed in the head of the instrument, the mirror bends the path of light at right angles to the axis of the handle, so that the beam projects from the head of the instrument.

- **Focusing sleeve**: The sleeve also varies the distance between the bulb and lens to allow the retinoscope to project rays that either diverge (*plane* mirror effect) or converge (*concave* mirror effect). Hence, the sleeve is also called the *vergence control*. In most instruments, the sleeve changes the focus (vergence) by moving the *bulb* up or down.

- **Current source**: This is provided by a battery in the handle (rechargeable or replaceable types).

Simply slide the sleeve of the instrument up or down to move the bulb. Moving the sleeve up creates the plane mirror effect; while moving the sleeve down produces the concave mirror effect. The Copeland instruments (by Stereo Optical Co, Chicago, Ill) use this system (Figure 2-4).

In other retinoscopes, the *lens* rather than the bulb is moved to change the vergence. This is also achieved by raising or lowering the sleeve.

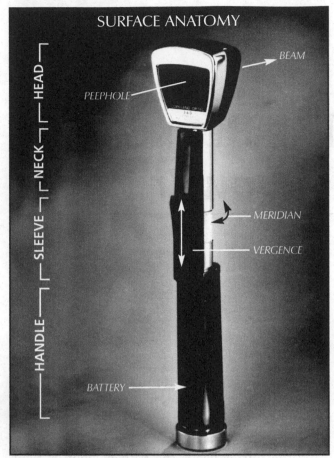

Figure 2-1. The external parts common to all streak retinoscopes.

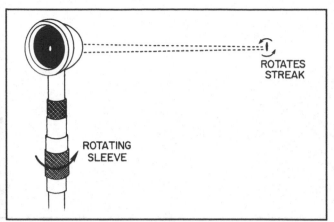

Figure 2-2. Meridian control. Turning the sleeve rotates the projected streak.

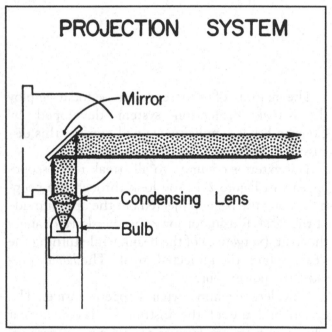

Figure 2-3. Projection system. Light path through handle and head.

Figure 2-4. Usual method of vergence control (lens is fixed) as seen on the Copeland type retinoscope.

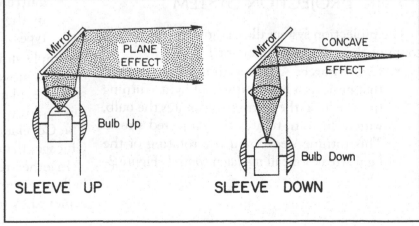

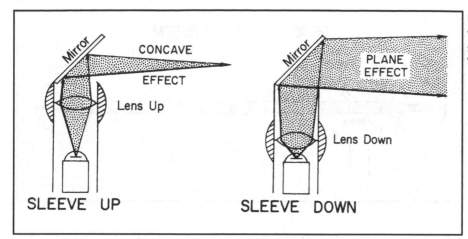

Figure 2-5. Alternative method of vergence control (bulb is fixed) as seen on retinoscopes made by Welch Allyn and others.

In all retinoscopes, you progressively increase the vergence of the beam from diverging rays (plane mirror), through parallel rays, to converging rays (concave mirror) as you move the sleeve from top to bottom (or vice versa).

As you can see by comparing the figures, instruments using a fixed bulb system work just the *opposite* from those with a fixed lens (sleeve up creates a concave mirror effect; sleeve down produces the plane mirror effect). The Welch Allyn, Propper, Keeler and other instruments use this latter design (Figure 2-5).

In all modern retinoscopes, the *sleeve* controls both meridian (streak rotation) and vergence (streak focus).

There is no need to understand plane or concave mirror effects at this point. You only need to know that the *plane mirror* simply acts like most familiar mirrors, reflecting parallel or divergent rays that never come to a focal point. The *concave mirror* converges rays to a point in front of the instrument, usually at about 35 cm (13 inches). From there, the rays cross and diverge (see Chapter 1, Figure 1-1).

Throughout this book, we will use the *plane* mirror effect unless otherwise specified. With the original Bausch & Lomb Copeland and Copeland-Optec instruments, this means *sleeve up*. Since these instruments are in widest use, you will be admonished periodically to "keep the sleeve up!" With the Welch Allyn and other instruments, keep the sleeve down. You will encounter no difficulty using these instruments for the exercises in this manual, once you are accustomed to *reversing* the position and movement of the sleeve. It is easy to

tell which focusing system your retinoscope has. Simply note whether the filament comes to a focus on your hand a foot away (concave mirror) when the sleeve is *down*, as in the Copeland instruments, or when the sleeve is up (Welch Allyn and others).

> The projection system is simple; the retinoscope emits rays of light that illuminate the retina (more precisely, the pigment epithelium and choroid). By turning the sleeve you can rotate the projected streak, and by raising or lowering the sleeve you can make the rays divergent or convergent.

OBSERVATION SYSTEM

The observation system (Figure 2-6) allows you to see the retinal reflex. Some of the light reflected by the illuminated retina enters the retinoscope, passes through an aperture in the mirror,* and out the peephole at the rear of the head. Thus, you see the retinal reflex through the peephole. When you wiggle the scope while looking through the peephole, you can observe movement of the streak you are projecting on the retina. Naturally, these rays emerging from the retina pass through and are acted upon by the optical components of the eye. The manner in which these returning rays are *affected* tells you about the optics of the patient's eye.

This is an optical aperture; the central silvering of the mirror is absent. Some models use a semi-silvered (beam splitter) surface to accomplish the same purpose. There are advantages to each system.

Figure 2-6. Observation system. Light path from patient's retina, through mirror, to observer's retina.

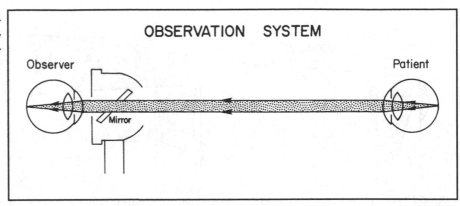

> By observing characteristics of the moving retinal reflex, you can detect refractive errors, such as myopia, hyperopia, and astigmatism. You then measure these conditions by placing lenses in the path of the observed reflex. When your correcting lenses create a situation known as neutrality, the power of the lenses is the measure of the refractive error.

HANDLING THE RETINOSCOPE

You will naturally feel most comfortable holding the retinoscope in your dominant hand, while sighting through the peephole with your dominant eye. This usually means right hand/right eye. While it is acceptable to start this way, I will periodically urge you to use your left eye (and left hand) for retinoscopy. Skill in using the retinoscope with either eye is invaluable and has important clinical implications we will discuss later. Once you are familiar with your instrument, force yourself to use your nondominant eye at least half the time—it is easier to learn good technique at the outset, rather than to correct bad habits later.

It is important to keep *both* your eyes open. Your natural inclination to squeeze the left eye shut while scoping with the right will not only prove fatiguing, but induces a temporary blur. This is annoying when you change over to scope with your left eye. To aid in suppressing the image from your unused eye, keep the room lights dim.

There is some disagreement over whether the instrument should be held with one or both hands. Argument is unnecessary, for it simply depends on the method being used. For *neutralizing*, in which the sleeve height remains stationary, we use one hand for holding the scope and rotating the sleeve. For *estimating* with Copeland's *spiraling* technique (which requires simultaneous vertical and rotary movements of the sleeve), we use two hands (see Chapter 9). In the spiraling method, we hold the scope in the right hand with the *thumb* on the sleeve to control its elevation, while we rotate the sleeve with the left hand (Figure 2-7A).

Retinoscopists who do not often use estimating techniques usually hold the instrument in one hand. The thumb presses the sleeve up (for plane mirror effect) while the sleeve is rotated with the index finger. With practice, most maneuvers can be performed with one hand (Figure 2-7B).

Copeland realized that most practitioners use estimation techniques only occasionally, so in his new model he designed a mechanism to hold the sleeve up. This simplifies one-handed retinoscopy for beginners, but it can be awkward to lower the sleeve when you learn more advanced maneuvers.

In this introduction to retinoscopy, we will emphasize plane mirror (sleeve up) technique. Inattention to sleeve height will induce error and confusion, so it is important to keep the sleeve up (unless, of course, you are using the Welch Allyn or Propper instruments, in which the plane mirror effect is achieved with sleeve down).

It is not easy to learn a one-handed technique, where you must hold the scope steady while rotating the sleeve. Once the knack is acquired, many novices are reluctant to train their nondominant hand in the same manner. The big advantage of this skill (with either hand) is that your other hand is free to change or hold lenses, while your arm measures the correct working distance (Figure 2-8).

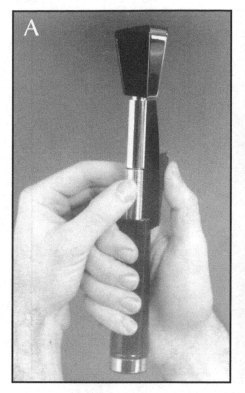 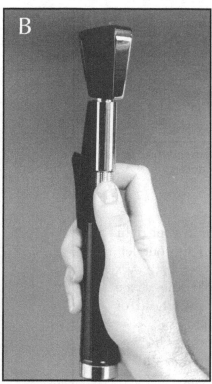

Figure 2-7. Holding the Copeland Optec 360 retinoscope. (A) The two-handed method for spiraling and (B) the one-handed method.

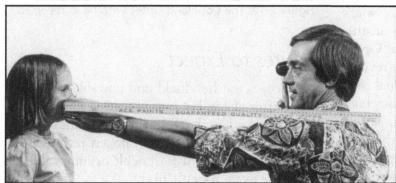

Figure 2-8. One-handed technique allows free arm to measure distance and place lens.

Ambidexterity and alternating ocular suppression are so important in clinical retinoscopy that you should adopt the habit of holding the instrument in your right hand while scoping with your right eye, and in your left hand when using your left eye.

The retinoscope should rest firmly against your brow or spectacle frame, so you can keep the retinal reflex in the peephole aligned with your pupil while you manipulate the scope. Resist the urge to close your other eye!

During retinoscopy, we observe the *movements* of the fundus reflex. In order to move the projected streak across the fundus, you have to wiggle the scope. The streak is always moved *perpendicular* to its axis. For example, when you place the streak axis *vertical*, you move it sideways. When you place the axis *horizontal*, you move it up and down (Figure 2-9).

You only need to move the streak a few millimeters across the patient's pupil, and you accomplish this by very slightly jiggling or rocking the scope. Remember to rest the instrument on your brow to avoid losing your view of the reflex. It is helpful to practice rocking your head up and down or side to side, while sighting through the peephole, as if you were nodding in agreement (or disagreement). Some examiners find it advantageous to rock their entire upper body.

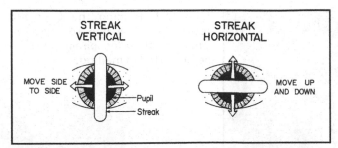

Figure 2-9. Movement of the streak perpendicular to its axis. The size of the streak is greatly reduced.

To summarize: Hold the scope in your right hand before your right eye, and in your left hand when using your left eye. Keep both eyes open and the lights low. Hold the scope against your brow and wiggle your head or trunk perpendicular to the streak axis.

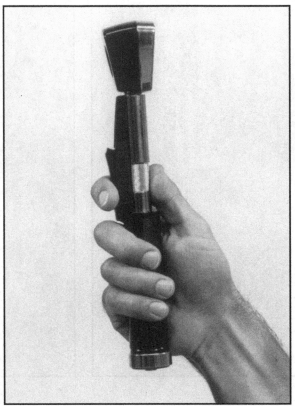

Figure 2-10. The Copeland Optec with head reversed.

THE INSTRUMENTS

After several years of puttering in his wife's kitchen, Jack C. Copeland finished a new instrument, which was marketed in 1968 as the Optec 360. This model incorporates a completely revolving sleeve held up by a spring and detent, dual controls for meridian and vergence, a pin-base bulb that cannot loosen, wireless connections, and a rechargeable capsule in the handle. All this was achieved at a cost of greater bulk. Copeland loved his improved model, but many who learned with the original version do not share his enthusiasm.

Many students find the Optec easier to use when the head is turned to reverse its position. You can do this simply by twisting the head around, which will place the rotary sleeve in a more natural position against your thumb (Figure 2-10).

In Figure 2-11, we have illustrated popular streak retinoscopes. These retinoscopes are all available with rechargeable handles, in which case you will need a battery charger (except when the Welch Allyn wall plug rechargeable handle can be used). Some of these handle adaptations were not anticipated by the designers of the instruments and adversely affect the balance and handling.

Features to Expect

All scopes are handheld and portable. All offer plano mirror effect, but not all feature full concave mirror effect. The latter makes neutralization of high myopic patients easier. Halogen retinoscopes are better used when it is difficult or impossible to darken the exam room lights.

Stereo Optical (Optec), Welch Allyn, and Heine retinoscopes have polarizing filters that will reduce the amount of glare you can get from reflections. Keeler claims to have a brilliant halogen illumination that will do up to 600 lux. Propper's unique mirror design provides bright illumination. Welch Allyn makes a special pocketsize retinoscope that can be a convenience for hospital consults.[1]

Always turn your power off when you are not using the scope to prolong battery life, especially if you place it flat on the table. Overheating the bulb shortens its life and when the scope is horizontal, this causes the filament to bend, producing a distorted streak.

Retinoscopy takes skill and practice. Don't expect to become an expert overnight. The more you practice, the better you get at this fine refractive error assessment.

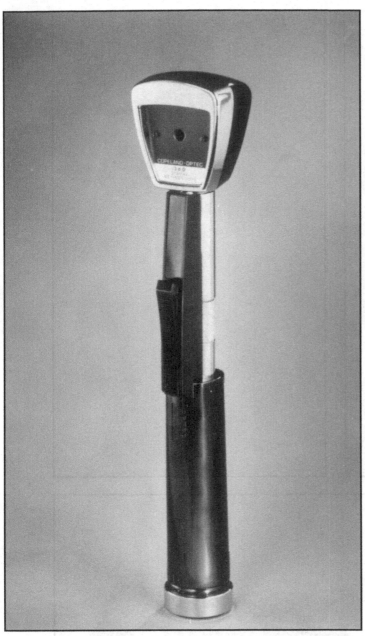

Figure 2-11A. 4v Copeland-Optec 360 Streak Retinoscope. Also available: 3.6 v Halogen Optec 360 Copeland Streak Retinoscope, 3.6 v Halogen Optec 360 Copeland Streak Retinoscope (with off-on polarizing filter that eliminates light reflections). Lightweight balanced handle. High-quality precision optics. Increased illumination for maximum output and shadow-free illumination. Extended battery life up to 20% providing greater flexibility and convenience. The entire head is adjustable for preferred eye alignment. Presbyopic lens assembles integrally into receptacle in head (optional) with a power of +1.25 D. Streak revolves 360 degrees without stops. Width of streak is controlled by smooth up-and-down action of the thumb slide. Improved electrical system in power capsule, no moving contacts to wear out. Each scope has plano mirror effect and full concave mirror effect, which makes ease for neutralizing high myopic refractive errors. Halogen or standard bulb models are available. Polarizing filter is available to reduce reflections (photo courtesy of Stereo Optical Company, Inc).

RETINOSCOPE MANUFACTURERS

Stereo Optical Company, Inc
800-344-9500
www.stereooptical.com

Welch Allyn
800-535-6663
www.welchallyn.com

Keeler
800-523-5620
www.keelerusa.com

Heine USA, Ltd
800-367-4872
info@heine.com

Propper Manufacturing
800-832-4300
www.proppermfg.com

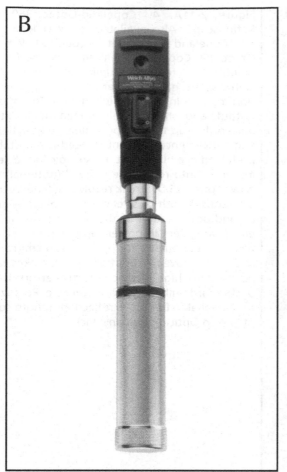

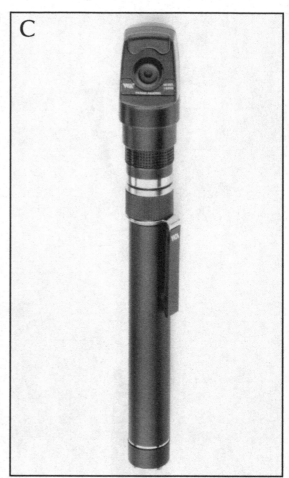

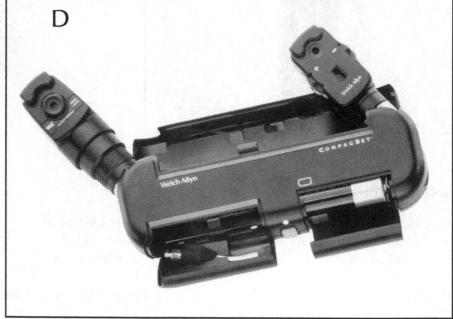

Figure 2-11 B, C, and D. Three Welch Allyn Retinoscopes. Figure B represents the WA-17200 Halogen HPX Streak Retinoscope; Figure C represents the WA-16200 Pocket Scope Retinoscope; and Figure D represents the 2.5 v Ophthalmic Compac-Set.

Included is an interchangeable bulb from spot to streak. An internal rotating sleeve improves maneuverability of the scope. A polarizing filter is available. It has a rubber brow rest, and magnetic fixation cards. The WA-17200 Halogen HPX Streak Retinoscope is said to be the brightest (photos courtesy of Welch Allyn).

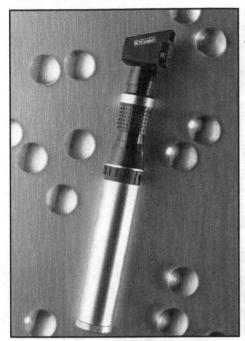

Figure 2-11 E. Keeler Professional Combi Retinoscope. This scope has continuous 360 degrees streak rotation, a choice of aperture mirror or semi-reflector viewing system, and brow or orbital rests (photo courtesy of Keeler).

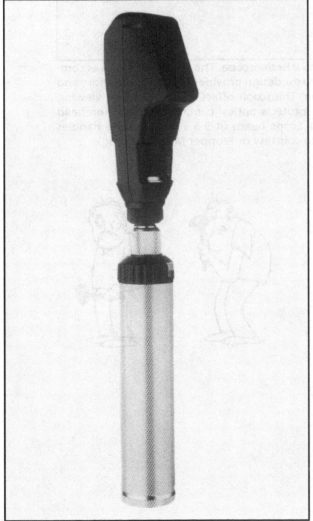

Figure 2-11 F. Heine 3.5 v Beta 200 Streak/Spot Retinoscope #C-02.15.353. This scope has a single control sleeve for vergence and rotation, and an integrated polarization filter eliminates internal dazzle and stray light. It also has 100% dustproof housing, and a HHL Xenon halogen bulb. Converts from streak to spot with bulb change and has a fixation card attached (photo courtesy of Heine USA, Ltd).

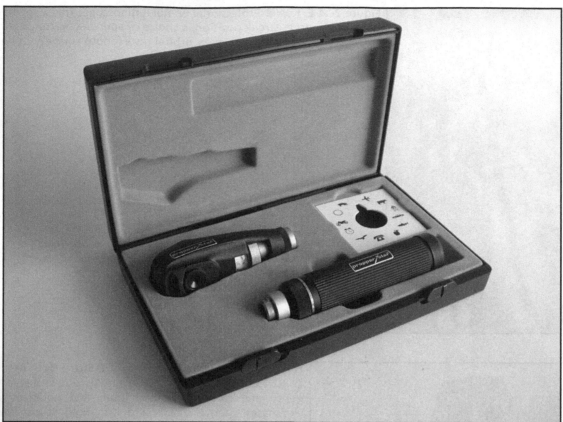

Figure 2-11G. Propper Star Retinoscope Set # 196900 3.5 v Retinoscope. The scope has features common to both streak and spot retinoscopes. Its unique mirror design provides bright illumination, and the multi-layer coating on mirror eliminates reflection. The scope offers a choice of two viewing apertures (2 mm and 4 mm), and a sliding dust cover protects optical components. Two forehead rests, including one for use with glasses, are included. Scope heads fit 3.5 v rechargeable handles that are either wall outlet or charging well type (photo courtesy of Propper Manufacturing).

REFERENCE

1. Norath D. Retinoscopes: The starting point of a good refraction. Available at http://www.visioncareproducts.com/12/retinoscopes.html. Accessed January 8, 2003.

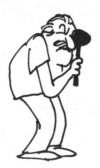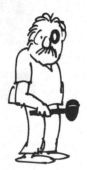

A REVIEW OF OPTICS

"The task I'm trying to achieve above all is to make you see."

D.W. Griffith, film director

In order for you to understand how we use retinoscopy to detect and correct refractive errors, we first need to agree on some basic terms; hence, this is a review of fundamental definitions. I purposely use no equations, so do not mistake what follows for a serious discussion of optics. References cited later explain the concepts in detail.

Read carefully and study the diagrams. This comes pretty fast!

REFRACTION

Light travels in *waves* like ripples on a pond. The *wavefront* consists of rays perpendicular to its surface. Natural light sources always emit rays that are *diverging*; we call this *negative vergence* (Figure 3-1A). When a lens *converges* light rays, we call this *positive vergence* (Figure 3-1B). The *curvature* of the wavefront depends on its radius; the further from its origin, the less the curvature. The wavefront from a source at infinity is so flat the rays are virtually *parallel*, and we say the wave has *zero vergence* (plano) (Figure 3-1C).

Diopters measure vergence. The curvature of the wavefront determines vergence, and we measure the curvature in *diopters* (D). The curvature or vergence varies *inversely* with the *distance* from the source (ie, the shorter the distance, the greater the

vergence). Since vergence varies (*inversely*) with distance, we can use diopters as a measure of distance. A wave *1 meter* from its source has a vergence of *1 diopter* (1 D). Vergence at 0.5 meter is 2 D. On the other hand, vergence at 2 meters is only 0.5 D, and at 6 meters is nil.

Diopters measure distance. Because we describe vergence as positive or negative, we do the same with diopters (note the signs for plus and minus in Figure 3-2). *Plus* diopters describe *convergence* and *minus* diopters describe *divergence*. For example, rays diverging from a point source have a negative vergence of one diopter (–1 D) at 1 meter; at half the distance, vergence is doubled (–2 D) (Figure 3-2A). Conversely, we can say that if parallel rays converge to a point focus in a distance of one-fourth meter, they have a positive vergence of four diopters of +4 D (Figure 3-2B). Thus, we can refer to a "1 diopter distance" (1 m) or a "four diopter distance" (0.25 m).

Refraction is simply the bending of light rays, altering their vergence. When rays pass unbent through a window pane, their vergence is unchanged; no refraction takes place. If rays passing through a medium do bend (refract), their vergence changes. Anything that alters the vergence of rays we call a *lens*. If a lens converges parallel rays, we say the lens has *plus* power; if it diverges the rays, the lens has *minus* power.

Figure 3-1. Vergence of rays from the source determines the curvature of the wavefront.

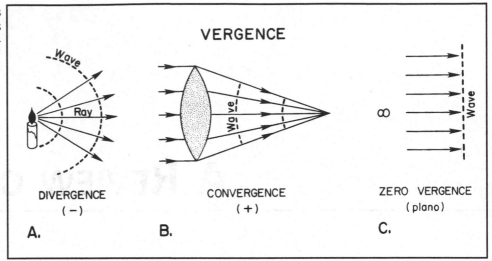

Figure 3-2. Diopters relate vergence and distance by defining curvature of the wavefront.

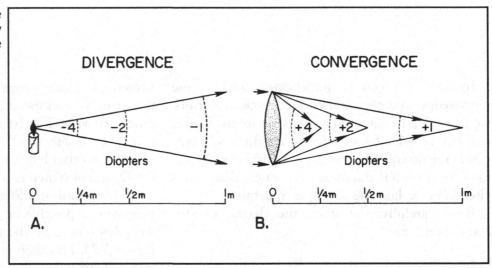

Diopters measure lens power. Just as diopters measure vergence and distance, they also measure lens power; that is, they describe the ability of a lens to bend light. The power of a lens is the *dioptric* distance of the focal point in meters. For example, a +1 D lens converges parallel rays *to* a point at 1 meter (Figure 3-3A).

Since dioptric power is the reciprocal of the distance in meters (ie, the shorter the distance, the greater the number of diopters), it follows that a +10 D lens *converges* parallel rays to a focus at 0.10 meter (10 cm). A –5 D lens imparts *divergence* of one-fifth meter (20 cm). Table 3-1 lists dioptric distances we use frequently in refraction. (You will notice that we refer to parallel rays; this keeps the calculation simple because their resulting vergence is simply that supplied by the lens.)

Table 3-1

Clinical Dioptric Distances	
Diopters	*Distance*
"zero" D	6 meters (20 ft.)
0.5 D	2 meters (6.5 ft.)
1.0 D	1 meter (3.3 ft.)
2.0 D	50 cm (1.6 ft.)
3.0 D	33 cm (12 in.)
4.0 D	25 cm (10 in.)
5.0 D	20 cm (8 in.)
10.0 D	10 cm (4 in.)
20.0 D	5 cm (2 in.)

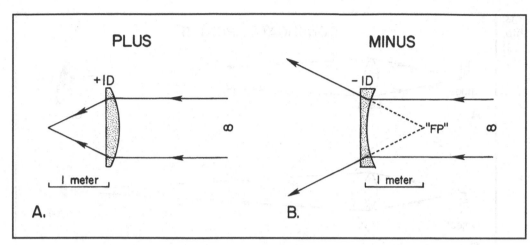

Figure 3-3. One diopter lenses: their effect on vergence of parallel rays. (A) +1 D lens converges rays to a point at 1 meter. (B) −1 D lens diverges rays as if they arrived from a point (FP) 1 meter from the lens

Diopters measure curvatures. The ability of a lens to bend light rays is related chiefly to the *curvatures* of its surfaces, especially at the air-lens interface. The degree of refraction increases *directly* as the surface curvature increases; a steeper curve (one with a shorter radius) refracts more than does a flatter curve. The final power of a lens is determined by both the front and back curves, but for the moment it is sufficient to remember that the *convex* front surface of the cornea produces positive vergence (plus power) on light passing through it.

In refracting light, the eye has the job of focusing the rays on the retina. The eye must exert considerable positive vergence on parallel rays to converge them to a focus on the fovea 22 mm behind the cornea. The plus power exerted by the human cornea and lens equals roughly 60 D.

REFRACTIVE ERRORS

Refractive errors (*ametropias*) have various definitions, from the familiar schoolbook diagrams of long and short eyes to the complex mathematical models of Gullstrand and others. Because optics has many ways of looking at the same situation (in terms of focal points, vergence, conjugate foci, etc), definitions of ametropias tend to overlap.

For our purposes, we will evaluate refractive error in terms of far points. The far point (FP) of an eye is defined as that point in space that is conjugate with the fovea when accommodation is relaxed.

Conjugate, as we use it in optics, means "corresponding to," and it is critical concept in understanding retinoscopy. When a luminous object is placed so that its rays pass through a lens to create an image on the other side, the *object* and the *image* correspond to (are conjugate with) each other (Figure 3-4A). Conjugacy demands reversibility of the relationship; if we now move the luminous object to the image point, the rays will pass back through the lens to focus at the previous location of the object, which we call the far point (FP) (Figure 3-4B). Thus we can measure the vergence of a lens from either side; if *we locate* the FP, for example, we will know the power of the lens.

We cannot easily study the power of the eye from within, but we can use conjugacy to measure the power from the outside. In retinoscopy, we rely on the reversibility of conjugate points in just this way; we illuminate the retina and locate the FP in space that is conjugate with it. Knowing the location of the FP, we know the power of the eye's optical system. Voila!

Returning to our evaluation of refractive errors, we ask: "Where do the rays focused on the retinal fovea come from?" If rays landing on the fovea come from infinity, we call this *emmetropia* (no refractive error). If rays focused on the fovea do not arrive from infinity, this is called *ametropia*. A corollary of the question is: "Where are rays from infinity focused within the eye?" Again, if they fall on the fovea, it is emmetropia, if elsewhere, ametropia. Let's examine specific examples to illustrate locations of FPs.

Figure 3-4. Conjugate points: (A) object-image relationship, where object is at FP; (B) reversal of conjugate relationship locates the FP.

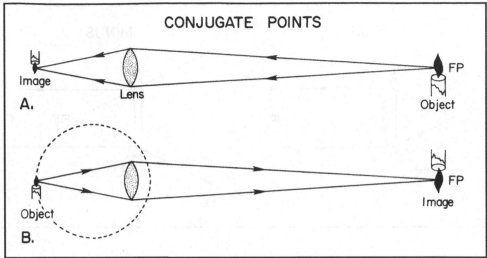

EMMETROPIA

Emmetropia means simply the absence of refractive error; parallel rays (from infinity) focus on the fovea. The retina is conjugate with infinity, so the FP of an emmetropic eye is infinity (Figure 3-5).

No lens is required to place the FP at infinity, so there is no refractive error. We say the refraction is *plano* (ie, flat) to describe a correcting lens of zero vergence.

AMETROPIAS

This category includes all refractive errors; parallel rays do not focus on the fovea, so the FP is *not* infinity.

Ametropias may arise from:

- Variations in the axial length of the eye
- Errors in curvature of refracting surfaces
- Variations in indices of refraction
- Shift in location of the lens
- Any combination of the above

The ametropias require a *correcting lens* to make the retina conjugate with infinity (ie, to move the FP to infinity). The *sign* and *power* of this lens define and measure the refractive error. It's as simple as that, and no math is required.

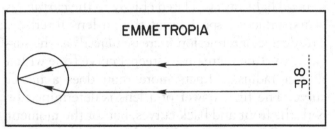

Figure 3-5. Emmetropia. Parallel rays focus on fovea.

SPHERICAL AMETROPIAS

If the refracting surfaces of an eye curve equally in all meridians (like the surface of a sphere), we say the eye provides *spherical* refraction. Parallel rays arriving at all meridians refract equally and come to a single focal point. In the spherical ametropias, this point is not the fovea.

Hyperopia

For any of the reasons listed earlier, a *hyperopic* eye has *relatively deficient refractive power*; that is, not enough positive vergence or plus power (Figure 3-6).

Parallel rays are not refracted enough and "focus" behind the eye (Figure 3-6A). The retina is conjugate with a point further than infinity, so we describe the FP as "beyond infinity"* (a virtual, not real, location; even optics requires poetic leaps of the imagination). A correcting *plus* lens converges incoming rays onto the retina. This makes the fovea conjugate with infinity, so the FP is now infinity (Figure 3-6B).

"Beyond infinity" puts the virtual FP of a hyperope behind the eye (in a circular universe).

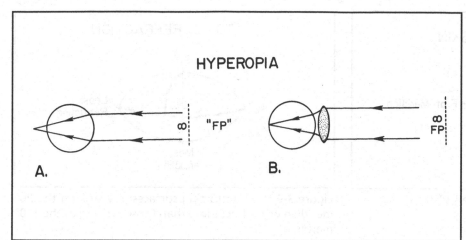

Figure 3-6. Hyperopia. (A) Uncorrected, with parallel rays focused behind the retina, and FP "beyond infinity." (B) Corrected by plus lens.

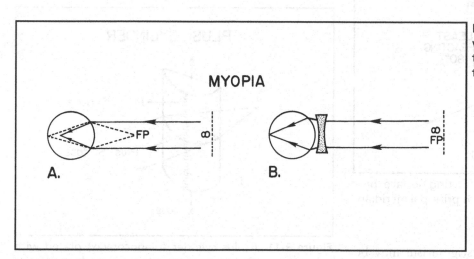

Figure 3-7. Myopia. (A) Uncorrected, with parallel rays focused in front of the retina, and FP closer than infinity. (B) Corrected by minus lens.

Myopia

As a consequence of the variables listed, a *myopic* eye has *relatively excessive refractive power*; that is, too much plus power (Figure 3-7).

Parallel rays are refracted too much and focus in front of the retina (Figure 3-7A). The retina is conjugate with a point *closer* than infinity, so the FP lies somewhere between the eye and infinity. A correcting *minus lens* diverges incoming rays back to the retina. This makes the fovea conjugate with infinity, so the FP is now infinity (Figure 3-7B).

ASPHERICAL AMETROPIAS

The refracting surfaces of the eye (especially, the anterior cornea) do not usually have the same radius of curvature in all meridians; that is, they are not spherical. In this case we say the refraction is

aspheric. Such a surface is called *toric* (or toroidal), and you can understand it best by imagining a section sliced through a football (Figure 3-8).

Since refraction depends on the surface curvature (increasing as the curvature increases), the principal meridians would refract rays differently. If the corneal surface were like that of the football, you can see that the *flatter* horizontal (180°) meridian refracts *least*, while the *steeper* vertical (90°) meridian refracts *most* (Figure 3-9).

Each of these principal meridians applies a different vergence, so there are two principal focal points in the eye. This defines *astigmatism*.

In Figure 3-10, note that the steep 90° meridian converges rays to the retina, while the flat 180° meridian (lacking sufficient vergence) refracts rays beyond the retina. We say the 90° meridian is *emmetropic*, and the 180° meridian is *hyperopic*.

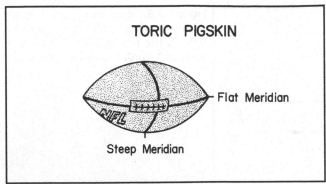

Figure 3-8. Sliced football as a toric surface.

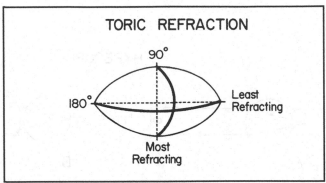

Figure 3-9. Toric refracting surfaces: ray striking the 90° meridian will refract more than those arriving at the 180° meridian

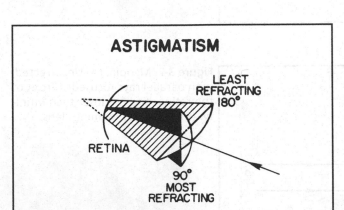

Figure 3-10. Astigmatism: toric refracting surface produces a different focal point for each principal meridian.

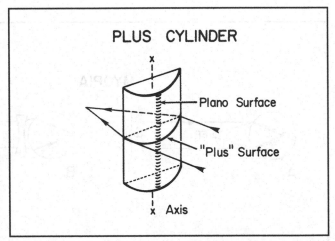

Figure 3-11. A plus cylinder (planoconvex) placed with axis vertical. Only the convex (power) surface refracts light. Rays arriving along the plano (axis) surface pass through unrefracted; the axis meridian has no refracting power.

The principal meridians in astigmatism may be myopic, hyperopic, or combined. An elegant classification looks like this (don't let it throw you):

- *Simple hyperopic astigmatism* (SHA). One meridian is hyperopic, the other emmetropic (as we saw in Figure 3-10).

- *Compound hyperopic astigmatism* (CHA). Both meridians are hyperopic.

- *Simple myopic astigmatism* (SMA). One meridian is myopic, the other emmetropic.

- *Compound myopic astigmatism* (CMA). Both meridians are myopic.

- *Mixed astigmatism* (MIX-A). One meridian is myopic, the other hyperopic.

We will examine each of these types in detail later.

We correct *astigmatism** with a lens called a *cylinder*. Cylinders may be plus or minus, but have their power only in the one meridian that is *perpendicular* to the axis of the cylinder. The *axis meridian* is flat (plano) and has no power (Figure 3-11).

The object of correcting astigmatism with cylinders is to *balance* the power of the two meridians in order to achieve a spherical refraction. When we correct astigmatism with *plus cylinders*, we want to *add* refractive (plus) power to the *least* refracting meridian. We leave the most refracting meridian alone. The cylinder is ideal for our purpose, since it applies power to only one meridian.

In a simple example of astigmatism resulting from a toric cornea, we would place the correcting cylinder *axis* (zero power) over the most refracting meridian, so that the *power* curve will lie over the least refracting meridian.

---

*For simplicity we are considering only regular astigmatism, wherein the principal meridians are perpendicular to each other. Irregular astigmatism, in which the major axes are not 90° apart, can not be corrected with cylinders. More on this later.

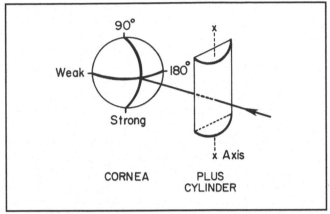

Figure 3-12. Correcting the corneal astigmatism with a plus cylinder. The axis is aligned with the most refracting meridian, so that power is added to the least refracting meridian.

In our football example with the flatter meridian at 180°, we place the plus cylinder *axis* at 90° in order to add plus *power* at 180° (Figure 3-12).

When we add power to the weak meridian to make it equal to the strong meridian, we neutralize the astigmatism and achieve a spherical refraction. We can then correct any remaining (spherical) error with plus or minus spheres as described.

> In summarizing refractive errors in terms of far points, you can see that if the FP is closer than infinity, we have myopia; if the FP is beyond infinity, it is hyperopia. The further from infinity the FP lies, the greater the refractive error. Spherical eyes have a single FP, while astigmatic eyes have two FPs.

CORRECTION OF AMETROPIAS

Now we can put all this together. Lenses alter the vergence of incoming rays and correct refractive errors, which in turn makes the retina conjugate with infinity (FP at infinity). The sign (+ or –) of the correcting lens *defines* the refractive error; the power of the lens *quantifies* the error. Diopters measure lens power by describing the vergence (positive or negative) that the lens applies to rays that pass through it.

Just as lenses are rated in diopters, so are the ametropias they correct. If a +2 D lens places the FP of an eye at infinity, the eye must be 2 D hyperopic. If a –3 D lens makes the fovea conjugate with infinity, the eye is 3 D myopic. Retinoscopy is based on this principle of finding the lens that places the FP at infinity.

We also use diopters as a measure of distance to describe the vergence of light waves. Rays from this page 40 cm from your eye arrive with a vergence of –2.5 D, so you accommodate (focus) your lens +2.5 D to put them on your fovea.

Conveniently, the diopter acts interchangeably as a measure of lens power, refractive error, vergence, and distance. An eye that requires a –4 D lens to place its FP at infinity is 4 D myopic; uncorrected, the FP is 25 cm—a 4 D distance.

Finally, diopters act as a measure of *corneal* refractive power based on the curvature. For convenience, we assume that a cornea with a 7.5 mm anterior radius has vergence of +45 D. So by convention, we use a dioptric scale (dropping the + sign) when measuring the corneal curves on a *keratometer* (ophthalmometer). When the keratometer reading of the meridians is 44 D at 180° and 46 D at 90°, it is easy to see that astigmatism is present and the vertical meridian is the most refracting. Consequently, we would expect a +2 D cylinder with its axis at 90° will add +2 D of *power* at 180, and correct corneal toricity. Note again that *axis* over the strong meridian places *power* over the weak meridian.

As mentioned at the beginning of this chapter, these are definitions, not explanations. I have purposely left much out, but if you have followed this so far, you are ready to proceed. If not, let Dr. Michaels[1] or Dr. Rubin[2] give you a hand.

REFERENCES

1. Michaels DD. *Visual Optics and Refraction, A Clinical Approach*. St Louis, Mo: CV Mosby; 1975: 201.
2. Rubin ML. *Optics for Clinicians*. 2nd ed. Gainesville, Fla: Triad Science Publishers; 1974.

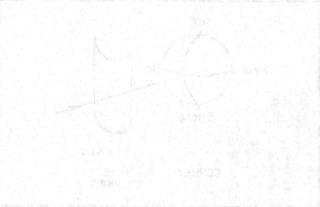

BASIC CONCEPTS

"If a man will begin with certainties, he shall end in doubts; but if he will be content to begin with doubts, he shall end in certainties."

Francis Bacon

LUMINOUS RETINA

As we have seen in the previous material, we will illuminate the fundus with the retinoscope and observe rays coming *from* the retina, as if it were luminous. When light leaves the retina, the optical system of the eye applies vergence to the rays. If we illuminate the retina with parallel rays (plane mirror), the reflected rays *leave* the eye according to the refractive error.*

That is:

- In *emmetropia*, rays leave parallel.
- In *hyperopia*, rays leave diverging.
- In *myopia*, rays leave converging.

This backward approach may seem confusing at first, but simplifies understanding of the retinoscopic reflex. Things happen differently when we illuminate the retina with rays that are not parallel, but we will ignore these for now.

In visualizing the situation, we will use a graphic presentation to illustrate luminous retina optics in three basic situations: emmetropia (plano), hyperopia (+1 D), and myopia (–1 D). Since the rays entering the eye remain parallel in all cases, we will ignore them entirely and simply look at what emerges. This is a very graphic presentation, so study and compare the diagrams carefully.

Figure 4-1 offers one more way of looking at the FP optics discussed in Chapter 3. We see the emmetropic FP at infinity, the hyperope's FP beyond infinity, and the myope's FP at less than infinity.

Now, picture yourself sitting before each of the eyes in Figure 4-2. Looking through the peephole in your retinoscope, you see these emerging rays as a red reflex in the patient's pupil. If you sweep the streak across the eye, the reflex you see will also move. If the emerging rays have *not* converged to a point (the FP), the retinal reflex will move in the same direction as you move the streak; this is called the *with motion reflex* (WITH). If the rays have come to the FP and diverged, the reflex will move *opposite* to your movements; this is the *against motion reflex* (AGAINST) (see Figure 4-2).†

Now picture yourself sitting almost at *infinity* looking through your retinoscope. This is what you would see in each of the three cases (Figure 4-3). In

---

*We saw the reason for this in Figure 3-4. By reversing the conjugate relationship between the FP and fovea, rays from the luminous retina are refracted by the eye to return to the FP.

†If you cannot control your impulse to try this, turn your scope on, push the sleeve up, and rotate the streak to a vertical position. Look at someone's fundus from about a foot away, as he or she gazes unto the distance. Move the streak side to side (perpendicular to the streak axis). If you see WITH motion (the retinal reflex moves with the face reflex), be satisfied and put your scope away. If you do not see WITH, put your scope away just the same and read on.

Figure 4-1. Rays from the illuminated retina. Correction refers to the lens desired to correct the refractive error.

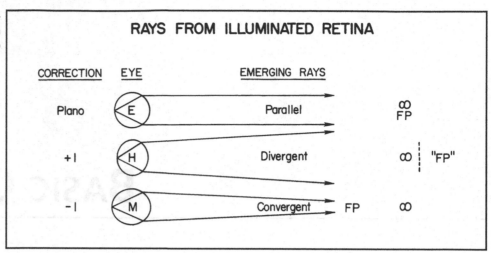

Figure 4-2. Retinal reflex movement. Note movement of the streak from face and from retina in WITH versus AGAINST motion.

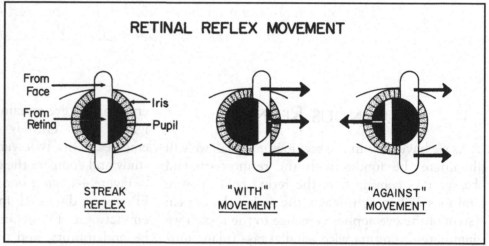

Figure 4-3. Retinoscopy at infinity. Note that within the FP, you see WITH motion; beyond the FP, you see AGAINST motion.

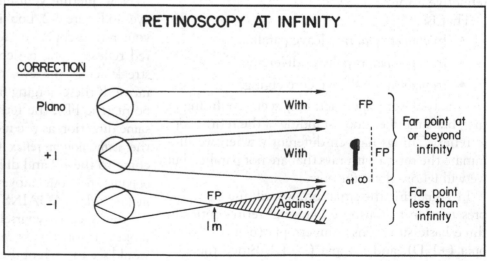

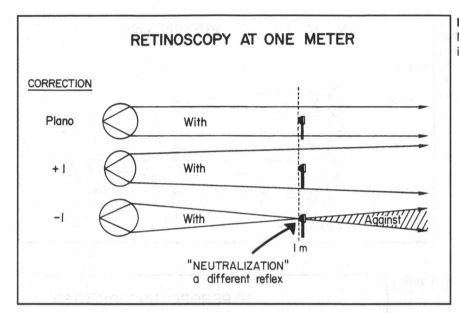

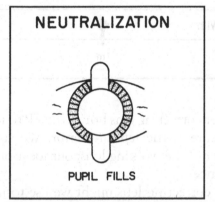

Figure 4-5. Neutrality reflex (NEUT) FP conjugate with the peephole of the retinoscope.

the emmetrope and hyperope, the emerging rays have not converged to the FP, so you see WITH motion. In the −1 myope, the rays have come to a focus at the FP (1 meter) and have diverged; thus, you would see AGAINST motion.

Consider this situation another way: if you see AGAINST, you are *beyond* the FP; if you see WITH, the FP is beyond you!

So much for what you would see if you sat at infinity. Optical infinity is anywhere beyond 6 meters (20 feet), but you cannot reasonably sit that far away: the reflex would be too dull, and you cannot place correcting lenses before the eye.

But if you sit at *1 meter*, the reflex appears brighter, and you can (almost) reach the patient conveniently (Figure 4-4).

With your scope 1 meter from the patient, you would still see WITH, but in the case of the emmetrope and hyperope, their FPs are beyond you.

However, in the case of the 1 D myope (FP at 1 meter), you would see a *different* reflex: if you leaned *forward*, you would now see WITH; if you tilted *backward*, you would see AGAINST. But when you sit with your retinoscope right at the FP of the eye, you see the *neutrality* reflex (Figure 4-5).

When you are at the FP, the pupil floods with light. There is no streak reflex and no movement WITH or AGAINST. The retina of the eye is conjugate with the *peephole* of the retinoscope. Since the reflex reverses itself (ie, changes from WITH to AGAINST motion) at the FP, some call neutrality the *reversal point*.

THE WORKING LENS

We have agreed that it is more convenient to sit closer than infinity. Yet, FP optics defines refractive error in terms of the *correcting lens that puts the FP at infinity*. How can we examine reflexes at infinity without actually sitting that far away?

You can stimulate infinity at any distance by placing a *working lens* before the eye. The power of this lens must equal your dioptric distance from the patient. The working lens makes your scope as if it were at infinity. Why this is so does not concern us here; take it as another article of faith.

Figure 4-6. Retinoscopy at 1 meter with a +1 D working lens. Working lens has increased the vergence of all emerging rays. Note that the emmetrope now shows NEUT, which means the FP is the retinoscope. The working lens places you at infinity.

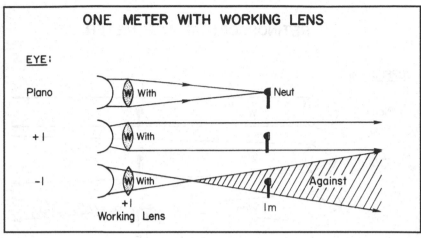

Figure 4-7. Hyperope uncorrected. WITH reflex indicates the FP is beyond you.

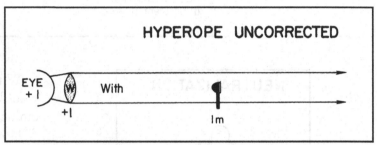

For example, if you sit at 1 meter, a 1 D distance, you would use a +1 D working lens before the eye to make it *as if* you were sitting infinity. Whenever the FP of an eye is conjugate with your retinoscope, it is just as if the FP were conjugate to infinity. So the working lens can move infinity up to any convenient working distance.

To see how this works, let's return to our exam at 1 meter, but this time with a working lens in place. Naturally, we would choose a +1 D lens.

If you compare Figure 4-6 with Figure 4-4, you will note that the reflexes we saw in the emmetrope and myope have changed. The reason, of course, is that in Figure 4-4 we viewed the reflexes from 1 meter, while in Figure 4-6, the working lens allows us to see the reflexes *from infinity* (even though our chair remains at the same spot). In all the diagrams that follow, remember that we see the reflexes "from infinity" when the working lens is shown.

THE CORRECTING LENS

Because the use of an appropriate working lens places you at infinity, you now need to find the *correcting lens* that will bring the FP to where you are.

Whatever correcting lens brings the FP to infinity is the measure of the *refractive error*. We can ignore the power of the working lens; our location cancels its vergence.

What correcting lens might we use to move the FP to you? Easy. Just recall that since plus lenses converge the emerging rays, they will pull the FP *toward* the eye. Minus lenses diverge and will push the FP *away* from the eye.

Now, let's take each of the cases in Figure 4-6, and see how we can measure refractive error.

We defined *emmetropia* as having the FP at infinity, with no correcting lens. In Figure 4-6, you see at the top that the FP is at your retinoscope (the working lens placed you at infinity). Therefore, the FP is infinity. Since no other lens was required, the refraction is *plano*. The reflex you see is NEUT because the patient's retina is conjugate with your scope. Neat and easy.

Now let's look at the *hyperope* (Figure 4-7). You are at infinity, and since you still see WITH, the FP is *beyond* infinity. Those eyes with a FP beyond infinity are, by definition, hyperopic. Hyperopes want *plus*, and plus lenses pull the FP in toward the eye, so let's add some plus. Try a +1 D lens for starters (Figure 4-8).

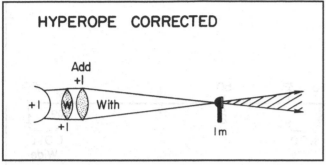

Figure 4-8. Hyperope corrected. A +1 D correcting lens has placed the FP at infinity, so the refractive error is +1D.

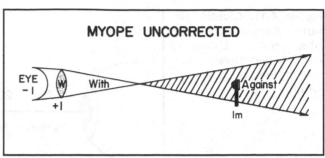

Figure 4-9. Myope uncorrected. AGAINST reflex indicates you are beyond the FP

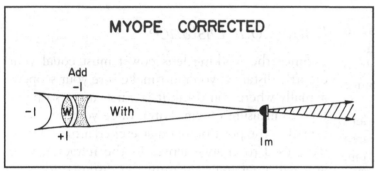

Figure 4-10. Myope corrected. A −1 D correcting lens placed the FP at infinity, so the refractive error is −1D.

Voila! Now you see NEUT. This means the retina is conjugate with you. You are at infinity, so the FP is now infinity. It took a +1 D lens to accomplish this, so by definition, the patient is a 1 D hyperope. Just like magic! (Ignore the power of the working lens.)

Now, on to the *myope* (Figure 4-9).

Since you sit in an AGAINST cone of light, you know the FP is in front of you. Eyes with a FP *closer* than infinity are by definition myopic. Myopes want *minus*, and minus lenses push the FP further out. So let's try to measure the myopia by adding a −1 D lens (Figure 4-10).

Now you see NEUT, so the retina is conjugate with your scope. Since it took −1 D to move the FP to infinity, the patient is a 1 D myope. Simple as that.

Perhaps you'd best run those by again. They are fundamental.

To Summarize:
1. The working lens (of power equal to your dioptric distance) makes your retinoscope as if it were at infinity.
2. The correcting lens that places the FP of an eye at infinity is the measure of the refractive error.
3. Neutralization (NEUT) is the reflex you see when the FP is at the peephole of your scope.
4. Therefore, the correcting lens that produces a NEUT reflex is the correcting lens for the refractive error (ignore working lens power).

THE WORKING DISTANCE

Now that you realize you can make *any* distance represent infinity (simply by choosing a working lens of the correct dioptric power), let's decide which distance to use. We will make a simple comparison of two working distances: 25 cm and 100 cm.

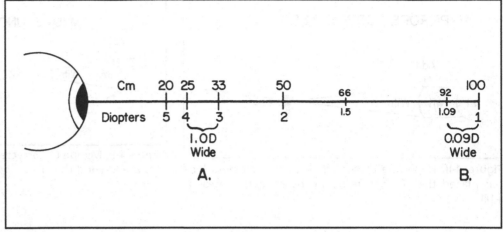

Figure 4-11. Dioptric distances. Compare the width of spaces A and B. Each is 8 cm wide, yet there is a ten-fold difference in dioptric width.

At *25 cm*, the reflex is bright, and it is easy to reach the patient, but the distance error is high.

At *100 cm*, the reflex is dim and it is difficult to reach the patient to change lenses, but the distance error is low.

What is this *distance error*, you ask. Well, let's assume you are sitting before the patient, prepared to perform retinoscopy at either 25 cm or at 100 cm, but you cannot precisely measure the working distance. For argument, let's say your estimate of the distance is off by 8 cm (about 3 inches). Now, compare these two locations on a dioptric scale (Figure 4-11).

As you can see, 8 cm (space A) is 1 D wide, while 8 cm (space B) represents only 0.09 D. Thus, if you worked at 25 cm, an error of several cm in estimating your distance can throw your results off by 0.50 D! Conversely, an error of equal magnitude is meaningless at 100 cm.

Since there are advantages (and disadvantages) to near and far working distances, most refractionists compromise by working at 66 cm (26+ inches). This is a convenient distance (roughly an arm's length) with a suitably bright reflex. And the dioptric value (1.5 D) is a nice round number. Since all refracting machines have a +1.5 D lens that flips in for retinoscopy, this has become a pretty universal working distance. We will use 66 cm, although some of you will find 50 cm (with a working lens of +2.0 D) more comfortable. In practice you will occasionally need to work closer to get a decent reflex from hazy media, or further away, to prevent a toddler from bursting into tears. Just be sure to choose the appropriate working lens. We will get into this later.

Know Your Distance

Since the working lens power must equal your dioptric distance, you must make sure your scope is actually where you think it is. First, use a string or tape to measure 66 cm. Later, once you are accustomed to the position of outstretched arm and bent wrist used to change lenses in the refractor, your arm will unerringly measure the distance for you. Do not fuss too much about the exact measurement; the beauty of this compromise distance is that an error of 5 cm (2 inches) in either direction is only 0.12 D (see Chapter 6, Figure 6-3).

Remember, too, that the working distance is a *reference point* for neutralization; you do not have to remain glued there. In the exercises that follow, you will need to lean forward and backward to confirm your observations, always returning to the working distance when judging NEUT.

We have chosen a working distance, and a working lens that makes that distance equal to infinity. Now let's get back in front of the patient and examine in more detail what we will see coming from the luminous retina.

THE REFLEX

Picture yourself sitting in the cones of light leaving the eye, viewing the retinal reflex through your scope (Figure 4-12).

When confronted with any reflex, you must first decide whether it is WITH or AGAINST. The location of the FP relative to your eye determines this; that is, the FP may be in front of you or behind you.

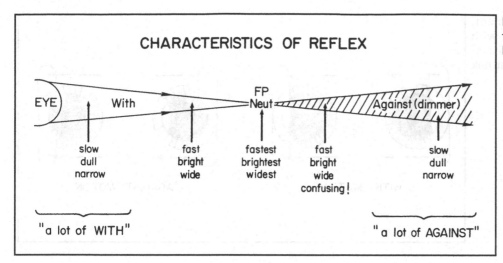

Figure 4-12. Characteristics of the moving retinal reflex on both sides on NEUT (FP).

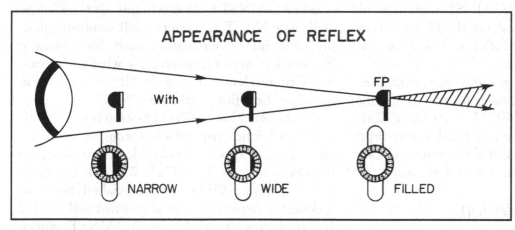

Figure 4-13. Appearance of reflex. Width of reflex at various locations in WIDTH zone. Compare with Figure 4-12.

Then, you need to judge the *amount* of WITH or AGAINST to determine how far you are from NEUT. Certain identifiable characteristics of the moving reflex will help you estimate your distance from NEUT. In turn, these help you decide how much correcting lens power you will need to move the FP to your retina. Experience in estimating will save much trial and error, and shorten your travel time to NEUT.

The moving reflex has three major characteristics:

1. **Speed**. The reflex moves slowest when you are far from the FP and becomes more rapid as you get closer. When you reach NEUT, the pupil fills, and no movement is seen. In other words, large refractive errors have a slow-moving reflex, and small errors have a fast movement.

2. **Brilliance**. The reflex is dull when you are far from the FP and becomes brighter as you

approach NEUT. Thus, large errors have a dull reflex, and small errors have a bright reflex. In our diagrams, AGAINST is cross-hatched because it is dimmer than WITH at any comparable distance from the FP.

3. **Width.** The band in the pupil is narrow when you are at a distance from the FP. It broadens as you approach the FP and fills the entire pupil when the refractive error is neutralized (Figure 4-13).

However, this characteristic is sometimes deceptive. When you are very far from NEUT, the reflex seems to broaden again in a kind of *pseudoneutrality*, which you will see in high error (that is, when you are a long way from the FP).

With practice, you will unconsciously use all three characteristics simultaneously to judge the *amount* of the reflex, so you can estimate how far the FP is from you. For example, if you see a lot of WITH motion, you would want to add a lot of plus

Figure 4-14. Reflex movement. Compare streak from face with streak from retina, both types of motion (the size of the face streak has been reduced).

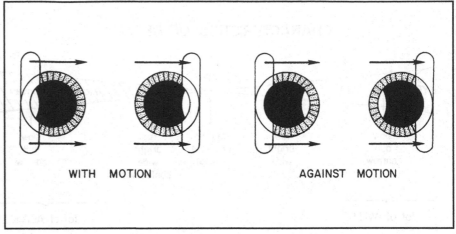

WITH   MOTION   AGAINST   MOTION

to pull the FP; a little AGAINST motion would call for a little minus to push out the FP toward you. Facility in estimating the reflex will save you a lot of time in changing lenses.

Now let's examine the reflex *movement* itself. There are several explanations for why the retinal reflex appears to move WITH or AGAINST the face reflex (also called the face band or intercept). Dr. Michaels explains it well if you want to look it up sometime, but don't get lost in that now.[1]

Avoid AGAINST Motion

Using AGAINST motion when neutralizing poses too many problems to make it practical, so plan to avoid using it. Look at the reflex once more (Figure 4-14).

In Figure 4-14, AGAINST motion looks a little contrary (as the name implies), and it is. The retinal reflex first appears at the side of the pupil opposite to the streak and moves in a *reverse* direction across the pupil, eventually disappearing at the side opposite the streak. For this reason, each of the three reflex characteristics is much more difficult to quantify on the AGAINST side of the FP. The *speed* of the reflex is difficult to estimate when it is moving in reverse. Since AGAINST is always further from the luminous retina, *brilliance* is reduced, making judgements difficult and margins fuzzy; in turn, this, makes it hard to see the *width* clearly.

As you will see very soon, the AGAINST reflex creates other problems as well. Moving opposite the streak, AGAINST motion is highly aberrated, especially near NEUT. It is often a dull, confusing muddle, difficult to evaluate, much less measure. Sometimes you cannot even grasp what you are seeing. One resident put it aptly: "If you can't figure out what the reflex is, it's AGAINST."

On the other hand, WITH motion is easily workable. It is bright, crisp, seldom confusing, and easily quantified. You will quickly learn to recognize degrees or *amounts* of WITH. WITH is agreeable, never contrary; WITH is dependable! So when seeking the refractive error, always first seek WITH. If you chance to stumble on AGAINST, quickly convert it by adding sufficient minus lenses to see WITH. A slogan might be "Stay with WITH and against AGAINST."

FINDING NEUTRALITY

To measure the refractive error with retinoscopy, we want to bring the FP to infinity (ie, to your scope when the proper working lens is in place). When the FP is at the peephole, you will see the NEUT reflex.

The correcting lens that accomplishes this is the measure of refraction. So the object is to bring the FP to you (to see NEUT, in other words), while you remain at the working distance.

How do you do this? Well, again picture yourself sitting in the cones of emerging light (as seen in Figure 4-12) with the FP somewhere in front of you or behind you.

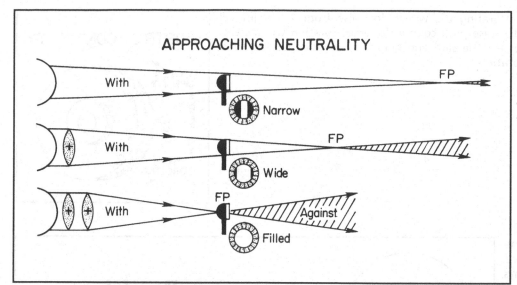

Figure 4-15. Approaching neutrality. Change in width of the reflex as NEUT is approached. Note that working distance remains constant, and FP is pulled in with plus lenses. Compare with Figure 4-13.

The *theory* is simple:

> If you see WITH, add plus lenses. When you see WITH motion, the FP is somewhere behind you. You would add plus to pull in the FP (to converge the emerging rays) until it reaches your scope, at which point you would see NEUT.

Let's look at it (Figure 4-15).

> If you see AGAINST, add minus lenses. When you see AGAINST motion, the FP is in front of you, so you would add minus to push out the FP (to diverge the emerging rays) until you see NEUT.

But in *practice*, it is so difficult to approach NEUT from the AGAINST side that we *overcorrect* to get the FP behind us. This will eliminate AGAINST and replace it with WITH; then we simply reduce the WITH until we reach NEUT. For example, if we see AGAINST, we might place –1 D lenses until we convert the reflex to WITH. Then, we would add plus (ie, *reduce minus*) perhaps in 0.25 D steps, until the reflex is neutralized. This approach from the WITH side is far better than

approaching the FP in minus lens increments from the AGAINST side. With this in mind, let's formulate some rules that will save you time and trouble. Watch closely:

> **Seek WITH , and follow it to NEUT.**
> *Rule 1.* If you see WITH, add plus (or reduce minus) until you reach NEUT.
> *Rule 2.* If you see AGAINST, add minus (or reduce plus) until you see WITH. Then follow Rule 1 to reach NEUT.
> *Rule 3.* Always use plane mirror (sleeve up) at working distance when neutralizing.

Be sure you understand the equivalence of the items above—adding plus power is the same as reducing minus, and vice versa. We are simply changing vergence. What you call it depends on your starting point; after all, it is a *direction*. If you are uneasy with this concept, pause momentarily to consider *dioptic continuity*. This is best illustrated by a lens power wheel, such as what you will use on your retractor or lensometer (Figure 4-16).

The principle of shifting the FP to our working distance is the same, whether we are neutralizing for myopia or hyperopia. Seeing WITH, we add *plus* power to increase convergence until we see NEUT.

Figure 4-16. Power wheel. Rotating the wheel clockwise from any point will increase minus power or decrease plus; counterclockwise rotation will increase plus or decrease minus power. The sign and numbers are unimportant; what counts is the direction of rotation.

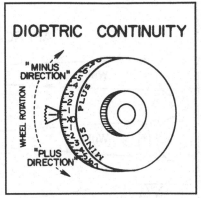

Figure 4-17. Neutral Zone. Spherical aberration produces a proximal FP 1 for axial rays, and a distal FP 2 for peripheral rays.

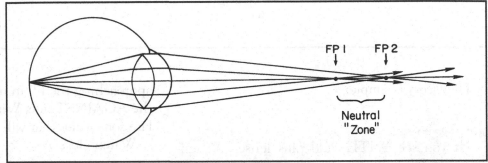

Figure 4-18. Doubt of neutral zone.

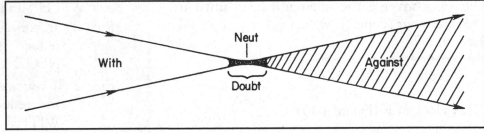

Seeing AGAINST, we add *minus* power to increase divergence until we see WITH, then reduce divergence until we see NEUT.

So WITH is the path to neutrality, which is our endpoint. The lens that brings you there is the measure of the refractive error.

INTERPRETING NEUTRALITY

Before getting a look at the actual reflexes, let's examine this all-important neutrality a little more closely.

Until now, we have considered NEUT as a point. Frankly, it is not a point but actually a *zone*, created by spherical aberration and other factors. The dimensions of this zone vary with pupil size and working distance (Figure 4-17).

The width of the neutral zone increases in direct proportion with the size of the pupil; it is narrowest with a small pupil. The eye in Figure 4-17 has no pupil, thus exaggerating the width of the zone. If you retinoscope with the pupil dilated, it is important to concentrate on the *central* pupillary reflex, ignoring peripheral aberrations.

The width of the zone also varies with working distance. It is narrowest when working up close, but this is not always helpful. If the zone is too narrow, precise judgment and working distance become critical. Minor inaccuracies produce major errors.

Within the zone of neutrality, there is considerable *doubt* about the nature of the movement (WITH or AGAINST?) the location (WITH in the pupil center, AGAINST in the periphery), and even the presence of movement (Figure 4-18)!

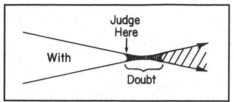

Figure 4-19. Judgement seat: NEUT is interpreted where zone of doubt begins.

When in doubt, stay in a little WITH.

REFERENCE

1. Michaels DD. *Visual Optics and Refraction, A Clinical Approach.* St Louis, Mo: CV Mosby; 1975;201.

To avoid all this uncertainty, and to stay on safe (WITH) ground, we make our judgement just *ahead* of where the zone of doubt begins (Figure 4-19).

Judgment of neutrality is an art, and its essence is to select a point slightly ahead of the zone of doubt, where there is *still* a faint central WITH motion. At that point, leaning *forward* a little will produce a definite WITH reflex. Leaning backward will first reveal uncertainty; then, further back, the confusing reflexes of early AGAINST.

Well, that's enough theory. We can now get down to seeing some of these things we have only described until now.

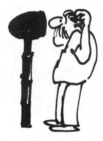

5

THE SCHEMATIC EYE

Now I would like to introduce you to the schematic training eye (or model eye), a mechanical device that simulates low spherical refractive errors and, with the addition of auxiliary lenses, also allows you to create higher spherical and astigmatic conditions. With the schematic eye, you use lenses to correct refractive errors just as in actual refraction.

The schematic eye has proved as useful and necessary to the beginner in retinoscopy as training wheels to a youngster on his first bicycle. As you acquire the basic reflexes, however, the once helpful crutch increasingly becomes an impediment to additional skills, and eventually you will cast it aside.

The schematic eye allows you to concentrate on detection and correction of ametropias—free of accommodation, shifting fixation, and drooping lids. The training eye has clear media and a wide pupil; it does not fidget, and it remains absolutely stoic. It also saves you from dealing with a crowd of people, because the training eye can duplicate a wide range of spherical and astigmatic refractive errors.

But, the schematic eye has many flaws, too: poor calibration, aberrations, reflections from auxiliary and neutralizing lenses, and phantom astigmatism. The skills necessary to handle a vigorous, fretful infant, or an older person with hazy media and small pupils simply cannot be learned from your cooperative training eye.

DESIGN

Basically, the schematic eye is a hollow cylinder (with two telescoping segments) that simulates the optics of the human eye.

The *anterior segment* contains the face (calibrated with meridian markings), pupil (sometimes of variable size), and the lens cells (to hold trial lenses for creating or correcting various refractive errors). Behind the pupil is a spherical lens of fixed focus, which simulates the positive vergence of the normal cornea and lens.

The *posterior segment* slides within the anterior cylinder. The back end is closed, with a red paper or retinal drawing to produce the retinal reflex. As this segment is moved in or out, the axial length of the eye can vary through a distance representing about 10 D. Pushing the posterior cylinder all the way *in* produces a short eye, usually equivalent to 3 to 5 D of hyperopia. Pulling the cylinder all the way *out* results in a long eye, about 5 D myopic. Graduated marks along the sleeve indicate the approximate refractive state. *Auxiliary* lenses placed before the eye create higher errors and astigmatism (Figure 5-1).

Figure 5-1. Basic design of the schematic eye (model eye).

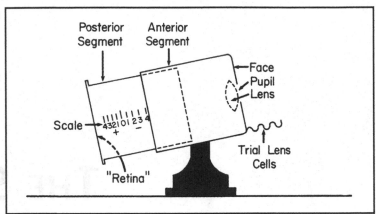

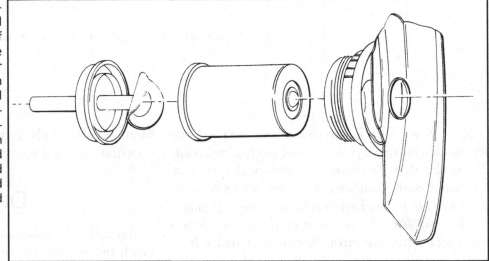

Figure 5-2. This schematic diagram illustrates an exploded view of the components of the homemade phantom eye as mounted on a phoropter face shield. Sequentially from left to right are the dowel passing through the film canister cap; the curved card representing the retina; the film canister with the lens glued over a hole in the bottom; and the milk carton top glued onto a phoropter face shield (Wessels).

Unfortunately, the dioptric scale is usually inaccurate, as a result of design, manufacture, and lack of prior calibration. Like bathroom scales, schematic eyes are usually *precise* (giving much the same result repeatedly), but not *accurate* (as compared to a standard). The eye may err by 1 D or more across the entire scale, but will produce reliable results once it is recalibrated.

Most teaching institutions have schematic eyes available on loan. In case you need to purchase one, I have included a list of popular models, along with some comments, at the end of this chapter. It is also possible to make your own[1] (Figures 5-2 through 5-4), which can be easy and fun.

Getting Started

Before proceeding, let's go over a few things you will need and some pointers in their use.

In the exercises that follow, you will find the useful life of rechargeable handles disappointingly short. If you do not have a corded instrument available, make it a point to turn off the scope whenever you pause momentarily and return it to the charger whenever possible.

In addition to your schematic eye and retinoscope, you will also need a *trial lens case* with a full range of plus and minus spheres and cylinders. Take a moment to familiarize yourself with the arrangement and markings of the trial lenses in the case (Figure 5-5A and B). Plus lenses are on the right half of the case and minus lenses are on the left. Spherical lenses are placed in the outer rows, cylindrical lenses in the center. All lenses have their sign (+ or −) on the handle and are often color-coded (in American sign code, *black* means plus, and *red* means minus; European coding is just the reverse). The dioptric power is marked on the handle. All beginners confuse spheres and cylin-

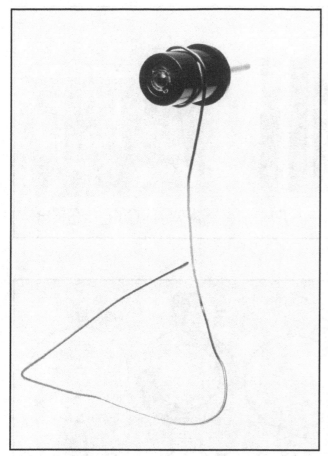

Figure 5-3. The homemade phantom eye is light enough to be independently supported on an improvised wire stand (made from a coat hanger) for refracting with individual hand-held trial lenses. Simply bending the wire adjusts the orientation. Placing a book or other heavy object over the base provides more stability. A more sturdy stand may be improvised by setting the phantom eye on a block of modeling clay, which can also hold trial lenses.[1]

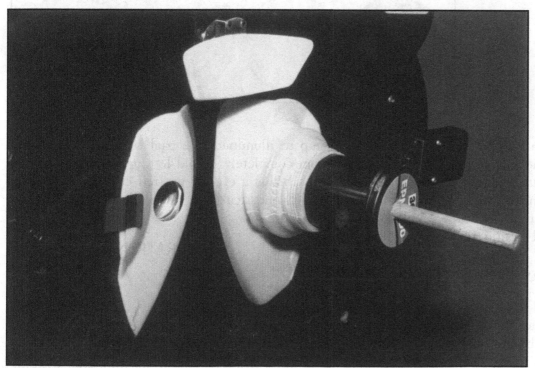

Figure 5-4. The home-made phantom eye is attached to the back of a phoropter face shield by means of a plastic milk carton top. This facilitates learning and performing retinoscopy without having to hold individual lenses in the hand. The degree of ametropia may be changed simply by moving the dowel in or out, and the astigmatic axis by rotation.[1]

Figure 5-5A. Trial case layout. On the left is a practitioner's set of corrected-curve meniscus lenses in color-coded mounts; note that minus cylinders are absent. On the right is a student set of plano-concave and plano-convex trial lenses, including minus cylinders, at less than half the cost.

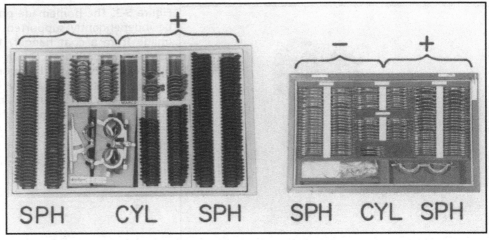

Figure 5-5B. Sample trial lenses. Top row: Plus spheres (1 and 2) and minus spheres (3 and 4); Bottom row: Plus cylinders (5 and 6) and prisms (7 and 8); note score mark on both cylinders and prisms—do not confuse them.

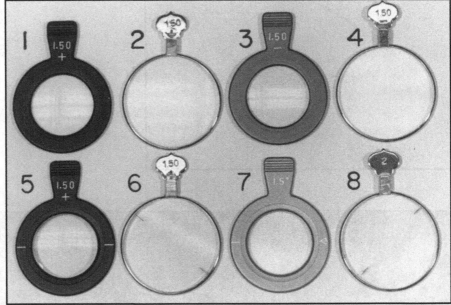

ders; the latter have a *score mark* on the lens and/or handle to indicate the axis. Watch for the mark; it is common for students to hastily confuse a +1.50 D sphere and cylinder in the dark, then spend an hour trying to understand the reflex they see.

Be careful to avoid mixing spheres and cylinders; get into the habit of putting each lens back in its place and you will save a lot of time fishing through loose lenses.

You will also need some uncluttered desk space, and a stack of books about 30 cm (12 inches) high.

The room should be semi-darkened to help you keep track of where you are aiming your streak (it is easy to lose), but not so dim that you cannot read the powers on the lenses. If possible, use a small

lamp to illuminate the trial case and darken the room completely. Avoid letting stray light fall on the schematic eye, or the reflections will confuse you. If your streak is not straight, replace the bulb.

CALIBRATION

Exercise 1

The schematic eye is simple to calibrate, and you will learn a lot in the process. To do this, you will need a +1.50 D sphere trial lens, your schematic eye, and a string or tape to measure your working distance (Figure 5-6).

Figure 5-6. Aligning pupillary axis of different training eyes to suit your gaze in a comfortable position at the working distance.

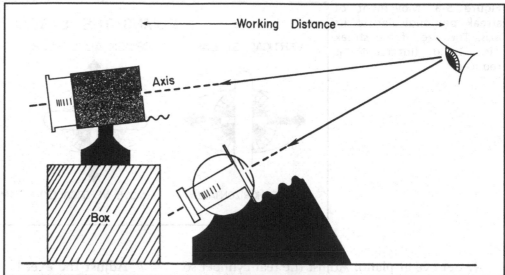

1. **Align pupillary axis.** It is most important to align your gaze with the pupillary axis of the schematic eye. Placed on the desk before you, most models lack sufficient upward tilt to allow you to look comfortably into the pupillary axis at the working distances. You may have to place the eye on a box or stack of books to bring it nearer your eye level. Unless you can comfortably align your gaze with axis of the training eye, it is impossible to maintain *optical alignment*; the resulting *off-axis* reflexes will really confuse your work (see Figure 5-6).

2. **Check optical alignment.** Hold the scope with the sleeve up in your right hand, viewing with your right eye, both eyes open. Sighting through the illuminated scope, you should see the two tiny light reflexes (Purkinje images, Figure 5-7A) from the lens surfaces. Keep these more or less superimposed to serve as a quick check of optical alignment.

   Remember that you are viewing *cones* of emerging light. These cones narrow rapidly near neutrality, and if you are a little off-axis, the reflex you see will be grossly incorrect. Make it a point to check the Purkinje images every time you pick up a retinoscope; alignment errors are *much* more costly than distance errors.

3. **Place working lens.** Place a +1.50 D sphere in the rear lens cell (closest to the eye).

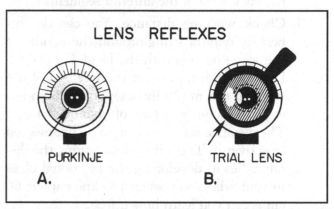

Figure 5-7. Reflexes from the schematic eye. (A) Purkinje images from the surface of the eye lens. (B) Trial lens reflections superimposed on Purkinje images. Note two reflexes, one from each surface of the trial lens.

Examine the lens reflexes. Ignore the red fundus reflex and look at the large, bright reflections from the surfaces of the working lens; their size and brightness depend on the surface curvatures. If you are troubled by great glare, the anterior lens surface is probably plano; turn the lens around and the dazzle should be reduced.

Notice how moving your position laterally or vertically affects the location of the working lens reflexes. Try to avoid these reflexes and concentrate on the tiny Purkinje images beyond them (Figure 5-7B). With practice, you will learn to displace and ignore these lens reflexes, while you keep the Purkinje images aligned.

Figure 5-8. Movement of streak perpendicular to its axis. The size of the streak face band (intercept) is reduced.

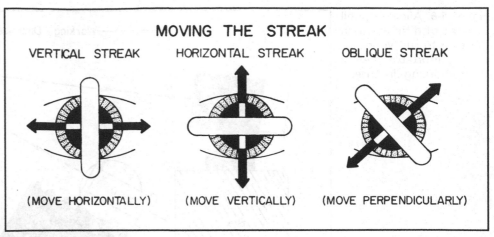

MOVING THE STREAK

VERTICAL STREAK   HORIZONTAL STREAK   OBLIQUE STREAK

(MOVE HORIZONTALLY)   (MOVE VERTICALLY)   (MOVE PERPENDICULARLY)

4. **Set eye at plano.** Adjust the rear cylinder so the zero mark on the graduated scale touches the back edge of the anterior segment.

5. **Check working distance.** You can do this best by tying a string around the handle of the scope just beneath the head. For our 1.5 D working distance, cut the free end of the string at 66 cm (26 inches); hold this end so it just touches the face of your model eye. The distance is not critical, so do not fuss too long over it. The value of measuring the distance lies in developing the positional clues in your arm—only when you know *where* 66 cm is can you learn how it *feels*.

6. **Check the reflex.** Dim the lights and align your streak at the 90° or 180° meridian. Rest the scope on your brow and wiggle your head (or trunk), making little sweeps across the pupil perpendicular to the streak axis (Figure 5-8). Try to keep both eyes open, while you locate the moving red fundus reflex.

   Now move in until you are about 10 cm from the eye, and note that the streak reflex in the fundus moves WITH your retinoscope movement. Now slowly withdraw from the eye, keeping this WITH motion reflex in view.

   Ideally, you should see neutrality with the sleeve up at the end of your string. When you lean in closer, you should see the WITH motion reflex. As you move back to the end of your string, this should broaden to flood the pupil at NEUT. Moving back beyond 66 cm you should see AGAINST motion.

7. **Adjust the eye.** If you do not see NEUT as described above at 66 cm, adjust the length of your model as follows:

   If you see WITH, lengthen the eye by pulling the rear cylinder out a little. If you see AGAINST, shorten the eye by pushing the cylinder in a little.

   A pearl worth remembering: pushing the rear cylinder in pushes the FP *away* from the eye, and pulling the cylinder out pulls the FP *toward* the eye. It will save time and confusion if you picture the FP located in front of you or behind you. When you see AGAINST, the FP is in front of you; you want to push the FP toward you, so push the cylinder toward you. If you see WITH, the FP is behind you; you want to pull the FP in, so pull on the cylinder.

   By thus manipulating the axial length in ever-smaller increments, you can shift the NEUT zone to 66 cm. When is it correct, you should see definite WITH when you lean forward 7 to 10 cm (3 to 4 inches). As you withdraw to the end of your string, this will broaden into a full, relatively immobile NEUT reflex (sometimes called "flooding out"). Judge the reflex at the pupil *center*; when in doubt stay in a little WITH motion. In Chapter 6, we will discuss refining neutrality and you may wish to repeat calibration. For now, be content with a rough estimate.

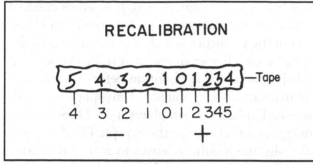

Figure 5-9. Recalibrating for a 1 D hyperopic error. Sleeve markings below are recalibrated by the tape scale above.

8. **Check the scale.** Once you are more or less satisfied with the situation, check the marking on the cylinder. If it is still at zero, you are unusually fortunate! More likely it will show an error of one or more diopters in either direction. This point represents the true *plano* state of your eye model.

9. **Recalibration.** If your schematic eye is in error by 1 D or more, you may wish to recalibrate it by placing a piece of tape over the numbers and correcting them. For example, if you found NEUT when the eye *showed* +1 on the scale, the eye is off by 1 D in the hyperopic (plus) direction. Corrected, it would look as shown in Figure 5-9.

   If the error is small (ie, less than 1 D) or the tape will not work, simply remember the correcting factor. You can make allowance for this when you create various refractive errors. For example, if your model eye showed NEUT about halfway between zero and −1 on the scale, this represents an error of about 0.5 D in a myopic direction. If you now wished to create a 2 D myopia in this eye, you would set the scale at about −2.5.

10. **Confirm calibration.** Now remove the working lens. Create 1.5 D myopia by pulling the cylinder out 1.5 scale units from your *corrected* plano (zero) reading (eg, if your plano was at a reading of +1, you would pull the cylinder out 1.5 units to about −0.5).

   Scope the eye: if your work has been precise until now, you should again see NEUT at roughly 66 cm. The reason you see NEUT from 66 cm at −1.5 D without a working lens

Table 5-1

Neutralization Table (66 cm)	
Lens Required to Place the FP 66 cm in Various Refractive Errors	
Scale Reading	**Neutralizing Lens**
−5	−3.50
−4	−2.50
−3	−1.50
−2	−0.50
−1.5	plano
−1	+0.50
0	+1.50 (*working lens*)
+1	+2.50
+2	+3.50
+3	+4.50
+4	+5.50
+5	+6.50

will be apparent from Table 5-1. If so, congratulations! If not, but it's close, this is quite acceptable, as the error may lie in your scale reading (ie, the point you extrapolate to represent −1.5 units). Remember, an error of one-quarter unit (0.25 D) will shift NEUT about 10 cm.

See if you can bring NEUT to 66 cm by a very *slight* shift of the cylinder. Be careful. A little shift goes a long way, which is another way of saying that this is a pretty exact technique.

If you are still way off, go back and start again: you are accommodating, off axis, or something else is awry. Do not proceed until you feel good about seeing NEUT when you are at 66 cm with no working lens.

11. **Check for astigmatism.** Now replace the original +1.50 D working lens, and set the eye at zero on your corrected scale. Recheck optical alignment and distance. First, use the vertical streak (90° meridian). Lean forward to see WITH, and lean back to your working distance to see NEUT. Are you still correct? If not, shift the sleeve a hair in or out.

   Now rotate the streak to the 180° meridian (horizontal); the NEUT reflex you see at string's end should be at roughly the same distance in both meridians.* If it is close, check the 45° and 135° meridians, always moving the streak perpendicular to its axis. By comparing these meridians as you lean forward 10 to 15 cm (4 to 6 inches), then back to the end of the string, you are learning a valuable technique called *meridional comparison*. If they all are about the same, your eye is roughly spherical (ie, it has no significant astigmatism). Just think, you can already diagnose the absence of pathology!

Some schematic eyes have the scale corrected so that no working lens is required at zero setting (WO-109).

Confirming Calibration

For those who desire to check the entire scale of the model eye (or the extremes at each end), the following lenses should produce neutrality at a working distance of 66 cm (see Table 5-1).

You should see from the table that the lens producing NEUT at 66 cm (the 1.5 D working distance) is always the algebraic sum of the refractive error and +1.50 D. The clinical implication of this may begin to dawn on you later.

By the time you have completed all this calibration business, you have learned a lot about retinoscopy, and you have already performed objective determinations of refractive errors. In succeeding sections, you may periodically need to recheck your calibration, as beginners commonly misinterpret the reflex in the early stages.

AUXILIARY LENSES AND VERTEX DISTANCE

We will use auxiliary trial lenses to *create* refractive errors greater than those obtainable by changing the length of the schematic eye. We call these *phantom* lenses, and they sit in the rack in front of the eye. These lenses create an ametropia of equal power but opposite sign; that is, *plus* lenses create a *myopic* error and *minus* lenses a hyperopic error. The power of the phantom is added to the setting of the schematic eye. For example, if you set the scale at –2 D and put a +10 D phantom before the eye, the combination would simulate a myopia of –12 D. The +10 D phantom simulates a 10 D myopia by converging retina rays to the myopic FP of 10 cm.

We also use auxiliary lenses to *correct* refractive errors, as you have already seen. To correct an ametropia, we add lenses of appropriate sign and power, with allowance for our working distance.

Problems arise, however, in creating or correcting errors when you stack several lenses together. The *nominal* power of a lens (marked on the handle) presumes a short *vertex distance* (the distance between the back of the lens and the front of the cornea). The effective power changes as the vertex distance (VD) increases. The difference is slight with weak lenses, but increases dramatically as the lenses become stronger.

As a rule of thumb, the effective power of a strong lens (±10 D) changes about 1% for each millimeter it is moved. The power of a 10 D lens moved 10 mm changes by about 1 D.[†] When you *increase* the VD, *plus* lenses get stronger (effective power increases) and *minus* lenses become weaker (effective power decreases). Since effective power relates to VD, make it a habit to keep the strongest lenses *closest* to the eye.

It is especially important to be aware of this change in effective lens power when working with the schematic eye, where the distance *between* the front and rear cells may be as much as 25 mm. Thus, on some models, the effective power of a strong lens changes by 25% when it is moved from the rear to the front cell. Obviously, you will want to keep the lenses close together.

However, errors will still creep in when using strong lenses, and failure to appreciate this leads to a lot of unnecessary weeping. Since the distance *between* cells is at least 5 mm, a –10 D phantom in the rear cell is slightly overcorrected by a +10 D

Be accepting of a little difference (perhaps 5 cm) for NEUT among meridians; nothing is perfect. If the FP differs by 8 cm (3 inches) or more between meridians (eg, NEUT is at 66 cm at 90°, but 58 cm at 180°) the model has at least 0.25 D of astigmatism (from the lens or retina) and will not work for your purposes. Check the paper retina to be sure it is flat and secure; if it is, the problem lies in the lens or its mounting. The phantom cylinder will drive you crazy; the eye is best exchanged. If this means returning it to the manufacturer, accompany it with a suitable note of indignation. Jack Copeland would be proud of you.

†This relationship (1%/mm) is purely coincidental, and is true only for the 9 to 11 D range.

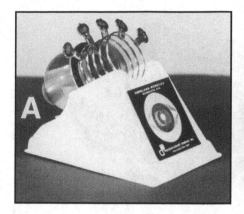
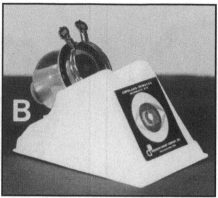

Figure 5-10. Replacing a stack of lenses (A) with two lenses of the same power (B).

lens in the next cell. With lens power less than +3 D, the effect between adjoining cells is insignificant. Thankfully, refracting machines have vertex compensation to prevent all these errors. You will only need to consider the VD of the machine itself (compared to the VD of the spectacles) in writing the final prescription.

As if this were not enough, each additional lens gives two more surface reflections for you to cope with. Each lens also reduces the brightness of the reflex, since the light has been refracted four times in the two-way path through the lens. Always use the fewest lenses to achieve a desired result; for example, replace a stack consisting of +1.50 D, +0.75 D, and +0.25 D lenses with a +2.50 D lens (Figure 5-10).

If you cannot borrow or make a schematic eye, Figure 5-11A and B and Figure 5-12 show some of the common models.

You will have problems with your schematic eye in the pages ahead; everyone does, but you will catch on. Be a little forgiving of its calibration and inconsistencies; it is imperfect, but it will teach you fundamentals. By the time you are truly thwarted by the model eye's limitations, you will be ready to retinoscope patients.

Since many of you may already be employed in an ophthalmic office, or have access to an eye refracting lane, I've asked Rich Reffner to explain his teaching method. He uses a refractor in retinoscopy of the training eye.

EYE LANE SETUP FOR RETINOSCOPY PRACTICE

Richard Reffner, COT

Typically, retinoscopy workshops are staged under less than optimal conditions. Meeting rooms are poorly illuminated—too dark to see engravings on the trial lens, or too bright for beginners to evaluate red reflexes adequately! Problems arise trying to find trial lenses in dim light. This is compounded by lenses that have been placed in the wrong sections of the trial case. Lenses may have become smudged from repeated handling. Further problems arise from drained or dead batteries or blown bulbs—with no replacements to be found!

Various authors have suggested an alternate method. One in-office method calls for using the refractor with a schematic eye secured to the headrest of the patient examination chair. The advantages of practicing retinoscopy with this method, rather than with loose trial lenses, are numerous. Refractor practice is more realistic, since you use the very instrument employed when seeing patients. Refractor lens selection is quick; you do not have to verify lens power before selection and there is less problem setting cylinder axis.

The disadvantage of in-office training when compared to a formal workshop is that you do not have the workshop instructor's knowledge and experience to help you. The service of a skilled retinoscopy instructor is paramount, if you are a rank beginner. Your sponsoring ophthalmologist or an ophthalmic medical assistant skilled in the art of retinoscopy may act as your mentor.

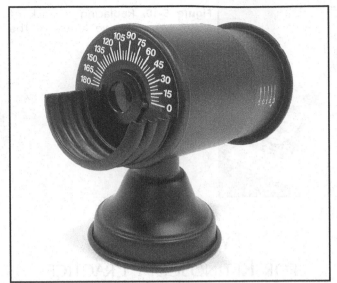

Figure 5-11A. Popular schematic training eyes. Schematic Training Eye WO-109. Manufactured by Western Ophthalmics, 19019 36th Avenue West, Suite G, Lynwood, Wash 98036, 800-426-9938. Corrected scale requires no WL at 66 cm.

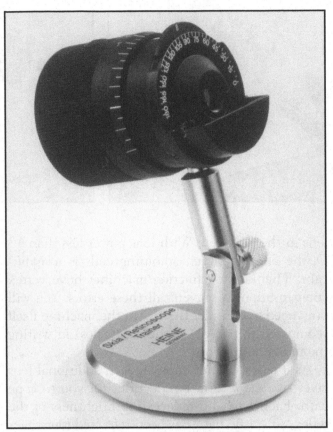

Figure 5-11B. Schematic Training Eye C-00.33.011. Heine USA, Ltd, 1 Washington Center, Dover, NH 03820, 800-367-4872.

A schematic eye such as the RTE (Retinoscopic Training Eye; Franel Optical, Apopka, FL) is required. The RTE (Figure 5-12) schematic eye is a good choice because it provides a base that has the rigid flat surface needed to firmly secure the schematic eye to the headrest of the patient examination chair.

The RTE can swivel vertically, and this feature enhances alignment with the refractor's aperture. Remember to check the optics of any schematic eye you buy. Schematic eyes with 0.50 cylinder or more are unacceptable, and should be returned for exchange.

Here's how to use the schematic eye in the exam lane:

1. Secure schematic eye to the headrest of the patient examination chair with a length of 3/8" Velcro strap (Figure 5-13).

2. Elevate the examination chair to a height that will position the schematic eye level with that of your eye.

3. Swing the refractor into place and align the optics of the schematic with the open cell of the right refractor aperture (Figure 5-14).

4. Be sure that the schematic eye is aligned as close to the back of the refractor as possible (Figure 5-15). Adjust spirit to level.

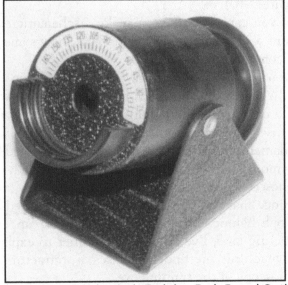

Figure 5-12. RTE (Schematic Training Eye). Franel Optical, PO Box 96, Apopka, Fla 32704, 407-884-1800 or 800-327-2070.

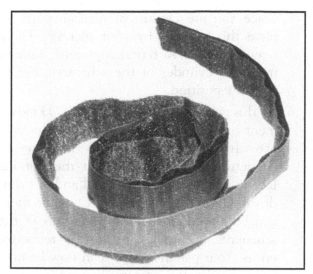

Figure 5-13A. Velcro strap.

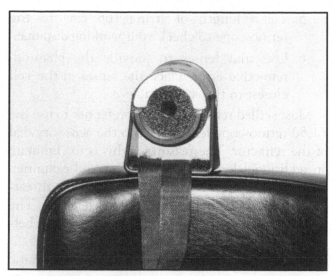

Figure 5-13B. Schematic eye secured to headrest of exam chair.

Figure 5-14. Swing refractor in place.

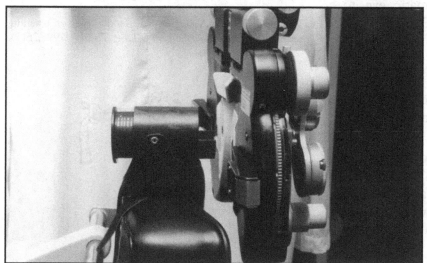

Figure 5-15. Be sure schematic eye is close to refractor.

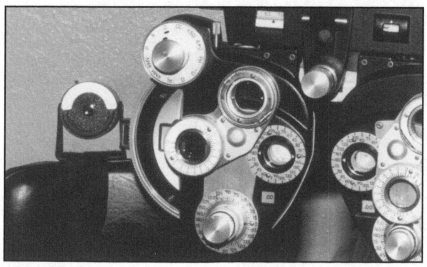

5. Tie a length of string (66 cm) to the retinoscope to check your working distance.

6. Use trial lenses to provide the phantom refractive error. Place the lenses in the cell closest to the schematic eye.

Most skilled refractometrists prefer not to use the +1.50 retinoscopy lens built into the accessory dial of the refractor. The reason for this is to eliminate an additional lens between patient and examiner, thus eliminating two refracting surfaces that threaten you with additional annoying reflexes. The fewer lenses between you and your patient, the better!

Next, check the calibration of your schematic eye:

1. Set the schematic eye at zero refractive error.

2. We will use the +1.50 retinoscopy lens to aid with calibration of the schematic eye to emmetropia.* With the +1.50 retinoscopy lens in the refractor and your streak retinoscope in hand, check the red reflex for neutrality when you scope it from 66 cm.

3. Adjust the cylinder of the schematic eye slightly in and out until a neutral end point is reached.

4. Check your reflex by moving to and fro slightly. Note WITH when you move toward the refractor (in front of the far point) and AGAINST when you move away from the refractor (behind the far point).

5. Once you are certain of neutrality, try to have this verified by your mentor. Then, remove the +1.50 retinoscopy lens. Tape or mark the cylinder of the schematic eye to hold the position.

6. At this point, you will observe WITH movement consistent with that of the emmetropic eye. In other words, this is how an emmetropic eye looks without the working lens in place. Various spherical and or cylindrical trial lenses, alone or in combination, can be placed in the trial lens cells of the schematic eye to create various refractive errors. Your patient's "eye" can now be neutralized, using the refractor lenses.

REFERENCE

1. Wessels IF, et al. A home-made model eye for teaching retinoscopy. *Ophthalmic Surgery & Laser Therapy.* 1995;26(5).

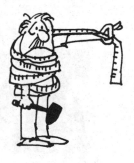

---

* *Emmetropia is the absence of refractive error. Parallel rays (from infinity) focus on the fovea. The retina is conjugate with infinity, so the FP of an emmetropic eye is infinity.*

6

SPHERICAL ERRORS

> *"Make thy two eyes... start from their spheres..."*
> William Shakespeare, *Hamlet* (I, v)

This section will combine lab exercises with our schematic drawings to help you make the transition from diagrams to actual retinal reflexes. Comparing your situation on paper with your actual location amid the emerging cones of light will help you to understand shifts in the far point as you apply correcting lenses; it will also help you to interpret the reflexes you see. In this chapter, we will use only *spherical** lenses (spheres), and for simplicity will omit the D from lens powers.

EMMETROPIA

Obviously, emmetropia is not a refractive error, but it is a good place to begin these exercises. Set up your model eye to maintain comfortable optical alignment at working distance. You may wish to recheck calibration before proceeding. If you have one of those schematic eyes that are very poorly calibrated, you may need to use a phantom lens to create certain refractive errors in these exercises.

For all exercises: Place the +1.50 working lens in the cell closest to the eye. If you are using the WO-109 eye (Western Ophthalmics), the zero mark is calibrated for NEUT at 66 cm *without* this +1.50 working lens. Make sure the sleeve is up on your

retinoscope; keep both of your eyes open. Dim the lights and then follow each step below, referring to the diagrams as you go. Each observation should be clear to you before you proceed further.

NEUTRALITY

Exercise 2

Now that you have "made friends" with your schematic eye, we will begin with a brief review of neutrality.

Adjust the eye to *corrected* zero (plano). Move in to check the reflex at about 30 cm (12 inches): it should be WITH. Move slowly back toward working distance, wiggling the scope perpendicular to the streak in any meridian. The moving reflex should become broader, brighter, and faster, until the pupil fills and movement in the pupil *center* seems to cease. This NEUT should appear when you reach the end of your 66-cm string. If necessary, make very slight adjustments of the eye to place NEUT at your working distance. Recall that pulling the cylinder *out* pulls the FP toward the eye; pushing the cylinder in pushes the FP away from the eye.

This should be your situation (Figure 6-1).

---

*Students frequently misunderstood this term. Recall that spherical refers to the refracting surface, curved equally, in all meridians like the surface of a sphere; it does not mean "round." A spherical eye may be oblong and a spherical lens may be square.

Figure 6-1. Emmetropia: NEUT at 66 cm with +1.50 lens.

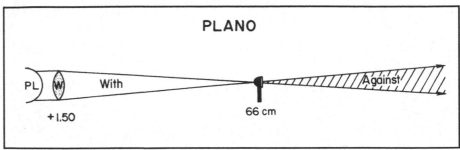

Move up to see a definite WITH, then recede slowly toward NEUT.

Move further back to see a clear AGAINST, then advance slowly toward NEUT.

Note that neutrality is easier to judge when approached from the WITH side.

REFINING NEUTRALITY

Exercise 3

While we have the schematic eye set at emmetropia, let's pause to review refining neutrality by shifting the FP or by shifting our position.

With your working distance fixed, you can shift the FP with *lenses*. When holding up lenses before the eye, make sure to hold them close to the working lens. Take +0.25 D, +0.50 D, –0.25 D, and –0.50 D spheres from the trial case.

Recheck NEUT at your working distance.

Hold up the –0.50 D lens and note a lot of WITH (minus lenses give you WITH by pushing *out* the FP).

Now alternate –0.25 D and –0.50 D spheres as in Figure 6-2, and compare the width and speed of the WITH band. Can you see the difference?

Now hold up +0.50 D and note AGAINST (plus lenses give you AGAINST by pulling in the FP).

Replace with +0.25 D and see less AGAINST.

Alternate +0.50 D and +0.25 D spheres and compare the reflexes.

It is hard to tell *degrees* of AGAINST!

At this distance, an increase or decrease of 0.25 D shifts the FP 10 to 14 cm in or out. Alternate the +0.25 D and –0.25 D lenses, noting again the effect on the reflex. Now, move to find the new location of NEUT with each of these lenses. It should be about like this (Figure 6-3).

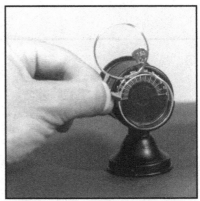

Figure 6-2. Method of holding two lenses so they can be rapidly alternated to compare reflexes.

Now put your lenses back in the case, leaving only the working lens in place.

Neutrality may be more precisely refined by small shifts of your *location*. Remember that interpretation of neutrality is imprecise, because NEUT is a zone of doubt (see Figure 4-19).

Examine the 90° meridian with your streak vertical. Approach and recede from the eye several times while observing the width of the reflex and the diffusion of its edges as you approach neutrality. Move in close enough to get a definite narrowed WITH band, then slowly recede while watching the band widen. Your natural tremor is usually enough to keep the reflex moving as you get near NEUT. After the pupil fills, note that there is still a little WITH wiggle in the pupil center. As you recede further, this WITH disappears into the reversal jumble we call NEUT, then AGAINST begins to appear. Do not go too far: judge NEUT when you can still see a little WITH in the center.

Rotate your streak to the 180° meridian (horizontal), advancing and receding to locate NEUT. Rotate your streak from one meridian to the other, comparing the reflexes. Are they the same?

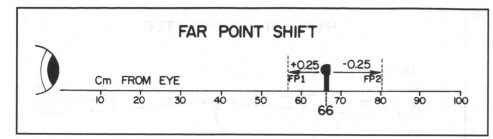

Figure 6-3. FP shift. Effect of +0.25 D (FP 1) or -0.25 D (FP 2) at 66 cm.

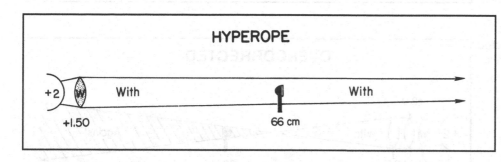

Figure 6-4. Uncorrected 2.0 D hyperopia, with working lens in place.

This advance and recede business proves an important habit to acquire. Remember that if you are near NEUT, you will always find WITH by leaning *forward* a bit. Do not let some odd AGAINST fool you. Always confirm your NEUT by leaning in to see a little WITH.

> Stay in a little WITH if not sure of neutrality.

LOW SPHERICAL ERRORS

In the following two exercises, the zone of NEUT may not be exactly at your working distance unless your eye is perfectly calibrated. Do the best you can. The object is simply to simulate low spherical errors and their neutralization.

Exercise 4: Hyperopia

Adjust your eye to simulate 2 D hyperopia by pushing the sleeve in to the corrected +2 mark.* Prepare −0.50 D, +1.0 D, +1.50 D, and +2.0 D spheres. Sleeve up, check working distance. Here is where you are (Figure 6-4).

Note definite WITH motion: the reflex band is of medium width. The FP is behind you.

Add a +1.0 D lens. See less WITH: the band appears slightly wider and faster (FP is moving in toward the back of your head, as in Figure 4-15).

Replace with +2.0 D. Do you see NEUT? Move back and forth to confirm. This is now the situation (Figure 6-5).

You must see NEUT here. If you do not have the FP at 66 cm, make a mini-adjustment of the cylinder to shift NEUT to your working distance so the following examples will be correct. (If it was way off, repeat the observations above, now that you have the eye better calibrated.)

Now, hold up a +0.50 D lens before the combination, noting AGAINST. This is an example of *too much plus* (Figure 6-6).

The eye is overcorrected, and the FP has moved in front of you.

Remove the +0.50 D and see NEUT. Flip it in and out, going from NEUT to AGAINST. OK?

Now, hold up −0.50 D before the combination, noting WITH. This is an example of *insufficient plus* (or too much minus) (Figure 6-7).

The eye is undercorrected, and the FP is now behind you. Remove the −0.50 D lens and see NEUT. Flip it in and out, going from NEUT to WITH.

Now put all of the lenses back except the working lens, which remains in place. Choose −1.50 and −2.0 spheres for the next exercise.

If your calibration is so poor that this takes you off the scale, use a −2.0 D phantom lens instead. For the combined +1.50 D working lens and −2.0 D phantom, you may substitute a −0.50 D sphere.

Figure 6-5. Hyperopia, corrected with a +2.0 D sphere.

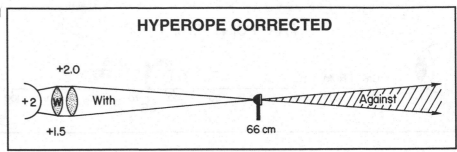

Figure 6-6. Hyperopia overcorrected by 0.5 D, showing AGAINST reflex.

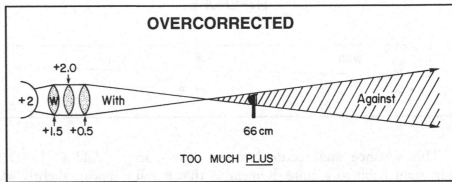

Figure 6-7. Hyperopia undercorrected by 0.5 D, showing WITH reflex.

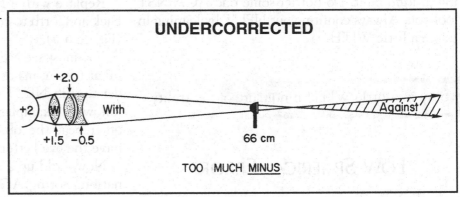

Exercise 5: Myopia

Adjust the eye to simulate 2 D myopia by pulling the cylinder out to your *corrected* −2 D mark* (Figure 6-8).

Note definite AGAINST: reflex band is of medium width. The FP is in front of you.

Add a −1.50 D lens. Note vague AGAINST, often a muddle (FP is diverging back toward you). The degree of AGAINST often becomes more difficult to judge as you approach neutrality.

Replace the −1.50 D with a −2.0 lens. You should now be seeing more or less NEUT and you can move forward and back to confirm.

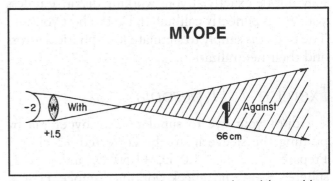

Figure 6-8. Undercorrected 2.0 D myopia, with working lens in place.

If calibration is so poor that this adjustment is difficult, use a +2.0 phantom lens instead. For the combined +1.50 working lens and +2.0 phantom, you may substitute a +3.50 sphere.

If NEUT is too far off your working distance now, make a microshift of the cylinder to place the FP correctly, then repeat this exercise.

Remove the –2.0 D neutralizing lens and take up the previous (–1.50 D) lens again.

Now flip the –1.50 D lens in and out, observing the reflex. When the –1.50 D lens is in place, you are seeing 0.50 D AGAINST; when you remove it, you are seeing 2.0 D AGAINST. Compare the two, and you should agree that smaller amounts of AGAINST are more difficult to interpret. This is why we approach NEUT from the WITH side.

You may now put all the lenses away except the working lens.

Exercise 6: Unknown Spherical Errors

Now we get to the fun! To avoid the confusion of inexact calibration of the model eye, we will create our unknown refractive errors with phantom lenses. While the phantom takes up space in your lens rack, this method limits the variables with which you have to contend. By using correcting lenses of equal power and opposite sign, we neutralize the errors created by phantom lenses. For example, a –2.0 D phantom lens creates a 2.0 D hyperopia, which we can neutralize with a +2.0 D sphere.

When creating your unknown, keep the power under +4.0 D, to avoid vertex power problems. Remember to minimize the number of correcting lenses by combining powers. In the eye models with only three cells, this is easy as you have only one left with which to work! Choose one meridian and stick to it for consistency.

Finally, to maintain interest, the phantom must really be *unknown*. Most trial sets have the power stamped on only one side of the handle, so simply turn it away from you. The color code (and sometimes the sign mark) is always visible, but this is unimportant. If you are in a group setting, have your partner or neighbor place the phantom; if not, just choose at random from the trial case.

Let's go. First, make sure your eye is at corrected zero. Place the working lens and recheck NEUT at your distance. Add a low *minus phantom* in the next cell.

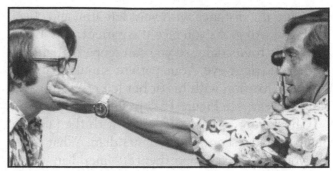

Figure 6-9. Retinoscopy through +1.5 D working lens held over patient's correction.

Study the reflex with both eyes open and the sleeve up. WITH or AGAINST? What sign do you place if you see WITH?

Add lenses in 0.50 D steps until you have NEUT near your working distance, then refine with 0.25 D steps. Stay in a little WITH if in doubt. Move forward and backward to confirm.

Now determine the refractive error (the power of your correcting lens). Ignore your working lens, and compare the correcting lens with the phantom. Are you close?

You should be within 0.50 D. If so, congratulations! Now put the lenses away. Remember to avoid cluttering up your space with loose lenses.

Now get out a *plus phantom* and repeat the same procedure. Remember to use enough minus to convert AGAINST to WITH, then reduce the minus to neutralize. Can you come within 0.25 D? If you have a problem here, it's usually with the initial zero setting of the eye. Recheck it.

Get a new minus phantom and repeat this time with your left eye, while holding the scope in your left hand.

Keep both eyes open! Watch working distance!

Keep at this, alternating signs and eyes, until you can consistently come to within 0.25 D of the phantom error, then take a break.

REAL RETINAL REFLEXES

Now let's try the real thing. Retinoscope your partner (or any handy, willing soul). Have your patient gaze at infinity, refractive correction (glasses or contact lenses, if any) in place, and hold your working lens before his or her right eye (Figure 6-9).

Measure the distance with your left arm, and check with the string. As you face the patient, you should be a little to his right, so you can scope his right eye with your right eye. Your patient should maintain distance fixation with his or her left eye gazing past your left ear (see Figure 13-3 in Chapter 13).

Check your optical alignment with the Purkinje reflexes. Now scope the 90° meridian. What reflex do you see? Next scope the 180° meridian. What reflex is present? Are the two the same? (If the reflex in these meridians is dissimilar, don't worry; we will come to astigmatism next.)

Repeat this drill with your left eye, scoping the patient's left eye while he or she maintains fixation with the right eye. Examine the location of NEUT in any meridian. Is it near your working distance? If not, what might you conclude for that meridian? Before concluding, be sure your patient's accommodation is relaxed and your alignment is correct.

At this point you should feel gratified by your achievement; you can now come within 0.25 D of the spherical refractive error. Perhaps you are right on the mark! Everything from here on is just a variation on the theme, so persevere; if you can do this much, you've got it made.

WORKING LENS

Before we begin retinoscopy in astigmatism, we need to go over some of the math so we can get rid of the working lens.

Until now, we have used the working lens in the rear cell, leaving the remaining lenses as the measure of the refractive error. Some refractionists do this with the refractor or trial frame, simply removing the working lens when retinoscopy is concluded. However, the reflections from the extra lens are annoying, and dim the reflex. With the schematic eye, the working lens occupies a needed cell and affects the vertex powers of the other lenses.

Since we are only talking about numbers, why not simply *allow* mathematically for the power of the working lens when computing the final refraction? Simply take the sum of all lenses after neutralizing, and *deduct the power* of the (absent) working lens.

Let's look at two examples. If you achieved neutrality at 66 cm with a total of +4.0 D before the eye, the calculation would be:

+4.00 D before eye achieved NEUT
−1.50 D *less* working lens power
+2.50 D refractive error

Likewise, if the final lens was +1.50 D, the calculation would be:

+1.50 D before eye
−1.50 D *less* working distance
  0.00 D refractive error

It looks simple, and it is. Try a quick example to prove it to yourself.

Exercise 7

Set the schematic eye at corrected zero with a +1.50 D working lens in place to check NEUT. Adjust if necessary. The eye is now emmetropic. Now *remove* the working lens.

Add a −1.50 D phantom.

Scope and see lots of WITH.

Add a +2.50 D correcting lens. Still some WITH.

Replace with a +3.0 D lens. See NEUT? OK.

Now let's look at what you have. The sum of the lenses before the eye is +1.50 D (−1.50 D + 3.00 D). This is called the gross power. From this, we subtract the working distance:

+1.50 D gross power
−1.50 D *subtract* working distance
  0.00 D refractive error

And wasn't the eye set for emmetropia in the beginning? It works!

Working Distance vs Working Lens

In the examples given, I slipped in the term *working distance*, instead of *working lens*. Since we chose the working lens *power* because of the dioptric *distance*, working lens power and working distance should always be equal. Therefore, they are (or should be) *synonymous*.

Thus, if you see NEUT with no lens (plano) before the eye at a 1.50 D distance, the calculation is:

0.00 D gross (at 66 cm)
 <u>–1.50 D *less* working distance</u>
–1.50 D net refraction

What is the point? Well, this lets you think in terms of distance and prepares you to use any distance. Let's say you wanted to work closer than usual, say at 50 cm. (What is the dioptric power of this distance?) If you needed a +4.50 D correction to see NEUT at that distance (2.0 D), the calculation is simple:

+4.50 D gross (at 50 cm)
 <u>–2.00 D *less* working distance</u>
+2.50 D net refraction

Got it?

Gross and Net

These terms *gross* and *net* should already be clear. The sum of the lens power before the eye is the gross retinoscopy finding. From this gross, deduct the working distance to find the net; this net is the true refractive error. Here are two more examples, using special distances:

+5.00 D gross at 33 cm
 <u>–3.00 D *deduct* distance</u>
+2.00 D net

–1.00 D gross at 25 cm
 <u>–4.00 D *deduct* distance</u>
–5.00 D net

If you come across a patient's chart with only a gross retinoscopy given, the 1.50 D working distance is implied.

In these examples, you will notice that because we deduct the working distance, hyperopes will always need *less* plus than your gross, and myopes will always need *more* minus in their final (net) correction. That may remind you of the neutralization table (see Table 5-1, p 44). Take another peek at it.

Getting Rid of the Working Lens

From now on we will neutralize without a working lens, as I hope you will do in practice. The disadvantages of the working lens should be apparent, and later on I will show you how its absence leads to a very nice method of subjective refinement, based on your objective retinoscopy.

Exercise 8

If you need to get more of a feel for handling these relationships, do the following:

First, recheck the zero setting of your eye with the working lens in place to be sure NEUT appears at 66 cm. Now, put away the working lens.

Have a helper create an unknown *hyperopic* refractive error of low degree by placing a –0.50 D to –1.0 D phantom lens before the eye. Check working distance. Do you see WITH?

Neutralize the reflex and determine the gross refraction.

To calculate net refraction, deduct your working distance.

Compare resultant power with the phantom. Were you more than 0.25 D off?

Repeat the above, using a low *myopic* unknown created by +2.0 D to +3.0 D phantom lens.

Review the relationship between gross and net in myopia and hyperopia to make sure that you feel comfortable with this before proceeding.

HIGH SPHERICAL ERRORS

There is nothing especially difficult about high refractive errors except their recognition. After you have detected and partially corrected them, these become small errors that you can already handle. For example, an aphakic patient (who had his cataractous lenses removed without implantation of an intraocular lens and wears +12.0 D spectacles) may initially confound you by the weird reflex he presents. Once you recognize the situation and place a +10.0 D sphere up before you start scoping, you will have a nice, recognizable WITH motion.

We are stressing recognition here because high sphere error is a great masquerader with two common disguises:

1. **Hazy media disguise.** This appears as either no reflex, or a very dull one. Placing *weak* plus and minus lenses without a change in the reflex seems to confirm your suspicion of opaque media.* When you suspect this situation, throw up *strong* lenses of plus or minus 5.0 or 10.0 D, to see if there is any change in the reflex. A definite, recognizable reflex will appear if it is a case of high error.

2. **Neutrality disguise.** This appears as a full, motionless reflex (pseudoneutrality), suggesting that you are near the endpoint. Simply lean in 10 to 15 cm (4 to 6 inches). If the reflex does not change, you *cannot* be near NEUT; try the strong lens check just described.

Let's try two exercises to develop your confidence.

Exercise 9: High Myopia
(simulated by a strong plus phantom)

Set the schematic eye at your zero, confirm NEUT with your working lens, then discard it.

Place a +10.0 D phantom lens in the rear cell.

Note the dull, odd reflex. High errors, especially AGAINST, are usually unfathomable.

Alternate +2.0 D and –2.0 D spheres before the eye, and note almost no discernible change with either lens.

Hold up a +10.0 D and note the persisting odd reflex, really dull now.

Hold up a –10.0 D lens. Ahh, recognizable WITH!

There is another neat method for unmasking high AGAINST, which we will describe later.

Exercise 10: High Hyperopia
(simulated by a strong minus phantom)

Use the same setup at zero, with no working lens.
Place a –10.0 D phantom in the rear cell.
Note dull, odd reflex. Do not confuse it with NEUT.

Alternate +2.0 D and –2.0 D spheres. Note minimal change with either. Can you see a hint of WITH when using the +2.0 D lens?

Hold up a –10.0 D and note the really minimal reflex.

Hold up a +10.0 D sphere. See recognizable WITH! Why is it not yet NEUT?

SPHERICAL ESTIMATION

To this point, we have remained at our working distance with the sleeve up. We always use this approach to determine the endpoint when neutralizing. Now we will introduce some changes in sleeve and distance to teach some useful shortcuts.

When you are confronted with a moderately high error, one showing a lot of WITH or AGAINST, it is helpful to be able to quickly *estimate* the refractive error, especially when you cannot change lenses rapidly (using trial frame or schematic eye), or with children, where cooperation is limited.

Refracting machines allow you to make *strong lens* changes so rapidly (usually in multiples of ±3.0 D), that trial and error often replaces skillful estimating techniques.

Learning estimating maneuvers at this point will get you comfortable with moving the sleeve and your body prior to embarking on retinoscopy in astigmatism. After you can handle cylinders, we will examine estimation again in more detail.

Before you can estimate the amount of the reflex, you must decide whether you have WITH or AGAINST motion. If you cannot interpret the reflex, try using a +5.0 D or –5.0 D lens, or more, to turn the confusion into a definite motion, then begin from there to estimate the amount of the reflex.

Assuming that you have a reflex to work with, but that it is broad, dim, and slow (suggesting a moderately high error), you proceed as follows.

Myopic Estimation: Far Point Location

If the reflex at the working distance is AGAINST, you are beyond the FP. This means that you have a myope of greater than –1.5 D. Recall that in myopia, the FP is relatively close to the eye; the dioptric distance of the FP from the eye defines the degree of myopia. From your working distance (AGAINST), move way in with the sleeve up until

---

By media we mean the transparent tissues of the eye: the cornea, anterior chamber, lens, or vitreous. Examples of opacities in the media reducing the retinal reflex are cataracts or vitreous hemorrhages.

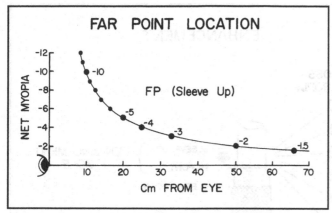

Figure 6-10. Estimating myopia. Distance of FP from the eye allows estimation of net myopia. Gross at 66 cm is determined by adding +1.50 to estimated net.

you find definite WITH, then ease back until you reach NEUT. This point, of course, is the FP, and an estimate of the dioptric distance will give you an idea of the *net* myopia (Figure 6-10).

You will notice that the dioptric distance narrows rapidly as the myopia increases, making FP measurement inaccurate in high myopia. Nevertheless, you can quickly tell –5.0 D from –10.0 D, thus saving yourself a lot of lens changes.

Remember that in myopic estimation, the FP location is *net* value, and neutralization would be performed with the gross. When going in reverse from net to gross, we *add* the working distance power (eg, the +1.50 D working lens factor) rather than subtract it. For example, if you found the FP at 25 cm (–4.0 D), you would expect NEUT with a –2.50 D lens at your working distance:

–4.00 D net (at 25 cm)
+1.50 D working distance (1.5 D)
_____
–2.50 D gross producing NEUT at 66 cm

Exercise 11: Myopic Estimation

Try it. The eye model should be at corrected zero with no working lens. Recall that you will see NEUT when the FP is at the *peephole* in the rear of your scope.

Place a +5.0 D phantom lens to simulate 5.0 D myopia. FP should appear about 20 cm from the eye. Does it? If you now place a –3.50 D lens, does the FP shift to 66 cm (–5.0 D net + 1.50 D = –3.50 D gross)?

Remove these and replace with a +10.0 D phantom. FP should be at about 10 cm from cornea to peephole, but it is hard to measure because the retinoscope head itself is 4 cm thick.

The technique has several potential errors, but the point remains—you can estimate myopic refraction by using the distance. Copeland had a far more precise method of locating the FP on a paper card in front of the eye. However, much of the accuracy is lost in the juggling of scope, card, and ruler, while little time is saved. Nevertheless, it is an entertaining exercise to try sometime.[1] Incidentally, myopic FP estimation is easier on real eyes.

Exercise 12: Confirming AGAINST

Before we leave myopia, let's look at an ancillary test that has nothing to do with estimating, but which frequently proves useful to beginners. Recall that with the concave mirror (sleeve all the way down with Copeland-type scopes) the rays converge to a focal point about 33 cm from the scope, then cross and diverge as they enter the eye (see Figure 1-1).

Inversion of the retinal image with the concave mirror produces a reversal of the motion. In other words, if the sleeve-up reflex is AGAINST, the sleeve-down reflex will be the opposite (WITH). This method chiefly has value when the sleeve-up reflex is in doubt. If you see a confusing reflex that might be AGAINST (often hard to judge), you can drop the sleeve and convert it to the opposite: WITH (which is always easy to judge). Try it with the +10.0 D phantom still in place, simulating high myopia.

Note that at 66 cm you can not decipher the reflex.

Drop the sleeve to see the *opposite* reflex. Is it WITH? This tells you that when the sleeve was up, you did indeed have AGAINST. Repeat the observation using a +5.0 phantom. The sleeve-up reflex is vague, the sleeve-down WITH is clear, confirming sleeve-up AGAINST. Thus assured, raise your sleeve again, and move in to find the FP (at 20 cm?) as described. Dave Norath expands on this technique in Chapter 11.

The converse of this test (that is, reversal of WITH when dropping the sleeve) is of no value because the WITH reflex is seldom confusing.

Figure 6-11. Estimating hyperopia. Appearance of enhanced retinal band and intercept in approximate degree of gross hyperopia. Note width of intercept at sleeve height producing enhanced retinal reflex.

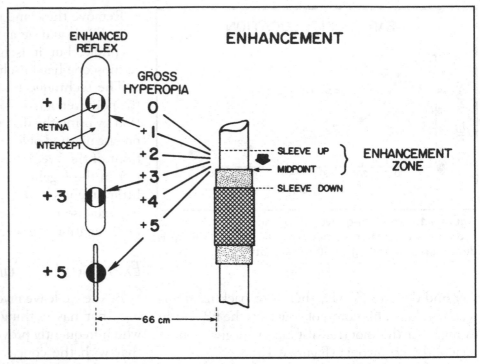

Summarizing estimation of myopia:
1. When in doubt, drop sleeve (sleeve-down WITH will confirm sleeve-up AGAINST).
2. Then with sleeve up, move in to find FP.
3. Dioptric FP gives net myopia.
4. Convert to gross (add +1.50 D), and place before the eye.
5. Check NEUT at working distance. Refine as necessary.

Hyperopic Estimation: Enhancement

When you see WITH, you can estimate the amount of gross hyperopia (up to about 5 D) by a technique called *enhancement*.

Slowly lower the sleeve at the working distance until you find the thinnest retinal reflex (the *enhanced* band). Compare this retinal band with the width of the *face* band (or intercept). The intercept is always enhanced with the sleeve about *halfway* down. These values are only approximate and vary a little among instruments; remember, we are only estimating!

At 1 D WITH, lowering the sleeve will not enhance the retinal band. In higher amounts of WITH, you can enhance the retinal reflex. As you slide the sleeve down a little more, the enhanced retinal band of 2 D WITH appears well before the intercept is enhanced. In +3 D, the reflex appears enhanced at a still lower sleeve height, nearer the intercept. The band of +4 D enhances just before the intercept. At 5 D WITH, the retinal reflex and intercept are enhanced with the sleeve at the same height. This technique is only meant for estimating gross hyperopia here. This is how it looks (Figure 6-11).

So if the narrowest (enhanced) retinal band coincides with the narrowest face band (intercept), you have about 5 D or more of WITH motion. Note that this is the gross power. Place this lens, then start again with the sleeve up. Slowly lower the sleeve once more to estimate the amount of additional plus required. This is easier to demonstrate than to describe.

Exercise 13: Enhancement

Set the eye at zero. Confirm NEUT with the working lens if necessary, then remove it.

Now, place a –4.50 D phantom, and see lots of WITH.

Figure 6-12. Estimating in children. Enhancement revealed at least +5 D, so the first lens chosen is a +5.0 sphere. Mother holds the lens, allowing you to maintain a nonthreatening distance.

Slowly lower the sleeve to produce the narrowest retinal reflex. Note that the enhanced retinal band and intercept occur at the same sleeve height, so you have at least 5 D of WITH. The sleeve is about halfway down, at the limit of the enhancement zone (beyond this, you will start to get reversal).

So, place a +5.0 D lens to correct this much WITH. Raise the sleeve up again, keeping the same distance.

Try to enhance the retinal band once more by slowly lowering the sleeve. You cannot enhance the reflex further, so the remaining error must be +1 D or less.

Add a +1.0 D lens. Do you now see NEUT at the working distance? (You should!) Calculate:

+6.00 D gross
−1.50 D distance
+4.50 D net

Note that net matches the phantom.

The chief value of this technique is estimating hyperopia in children. For example, if you initially found enhancement of the reflex and intercept at the same (+5) sleeve height, you would know there was at least 5 D of gross hyperopia. So the first lens you would pick up would be a +5.0 D sphere. Repeating the test through your hand-held +5.0 D would help you estimate how much more plus you would require. This saves a lot of tears, on both sides of the scope (Figure 6-12).

> **Summarizing estimation of hyperopia:**
> 1. If you see WITH at working distance, drop sleeve to enhance.
> 2. If you cannot enhance, it is +1 D (gross) or less.
> 3. If you can enhance, is it under +5 D or over +5 D?
>   a. If under, try a +3.0 sphere. Raise sleeve and begin neutralizing.
>   b. If over, place a +5.0 sphere, raise sleeve, and begin again to enhance.

This enhancement technique is much more useful in measuring residual WITH when neutralizing astigmatism, so we will see it again. If you need to know why this method works, ask the experts.[2]

Remember, lowering the sleeve or moving in are only maneuvers for estimation. Neutralization, as always, is performed with the sleeve up at working distance.

Now that you are expert in spherical errors, let's move on to more challenging matters.

REFERENCES

1. Copeland JC. Streak retinoscopy. In: Sloane AE, ed. *Manual of Refraction*. 2nd ed. Boston, Mass: Little, Brown, and Co; 1970:83,102,106.
2. Weinstock SM, Wirtschafter JD. *A Decision-Oriented Manual of Retinoscopy*. Springfield, Ill: Charles C. Thomas; 1976: 6,99.

ASTIGMATIC ERRORS

"But optics sharp it needs, I ween, To see what is not to be seen."

John Trumbull, *McFingal* (1782)

Before we proceed, let's review the optics of astigmatism to be sure we agree on some basic terms.

Astigmatism, as we saw in Chapter 3, describes what happens when light is not refracted to a single focal point. In an *aspheric* eye, all of the ocular meridians refract light differently, usually because the corneal surface is toric (see Figure 3-8). We call those meridians that refract the most and the least the *principal* meridians; each brings arriving rays to a different point (actually, a line) of focus at the back of the eye. Thus, there are two principal foci, and these may occur in front of, on, or "behind" the retina. We really do not care where they fall, for in retinoscopic FP optics, only the location of the FPs in *front* of the eye matters to us.

For now, we will assume that all ocular astigmatism results from differences in *corneal* meridians; significant astigmatism of the lens is uncommon and safely ignored (except when fitting contact lenses).

Ocular *meridians* are defined conventionally for both eyes in degrees from 1 to 180 as shown. Note that there is no "zero" meridian, nor any angle larger than 180°. The right eye is traditionally abbreviated OD (*oculus dexter*), the left eye OS (*oculus sinister*) (Figure 7-1).

In *regular* astigmatism, the principal meridians are 90° apart (eg, at 90°/180°). We can correct these with *cylindrical lenses*, which also have their principal meridians perpendicular to each other. *Plus* cylinders, with their axis (zero power) aligned with the stronger (most refractive) meridian, add power to the weaker meridian. When the correcting cylinder on the proper axis equals the corneal "cylinder," the meridians are balanced, astigmatism is neutralized, and we have created a spherical condition.

In *irregular* astigmatism, the principal meridians are not perpendicular, so they cannot be corrected with cylinders. (This unusual circumstance arises mostly from corneal irregularities.)

Oblique astigmatism (not to be confused with the irregular type) is simply regular astigmatism that is tilted. The meridians are perpendicular, but are at other than the usual 90°/180° configuration, for example, at 45°/135°.

Astigmatism "with the rule" refers to the axis of the plus cylinder standing more or less *vertical* (75° to 105°). "Against the rule" means the plus cylinder axis lies relatively *horizontal* (165° to 15°). These terms loosely describe the location of the *most* refractive corneal meridian (and the axis of its accompanying plus cylinder), which is generally erect in youth and supine in older age.

Figure 7-1. Standard notation for ocular meridians and axis of correcting cylinders, examiner's view.

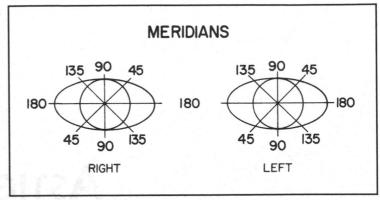

Figure 7-2. Appearance of astigmatic reflexes. NEUT is seen with streak at 180°: (A) while there is still WITH motion when the streak is rotated to 90°. (B) This is an example of simple hyperopic astigmatism with the rule.

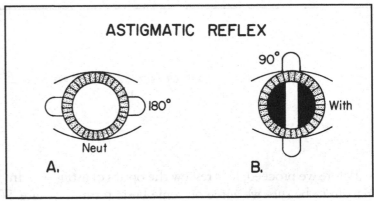

So, we usually find that "with-the-rule" astigmatism in younger patients often shifts over the years through oblique to eventually become "against the rule" in older persons.

We say a patient has *symmetrical* astigmatism when the axes of the correcting cylinders in both eyes total about 180° (ie, OD 100°, OS 80°). *Asymmetry* is not abnormal, simply uncommon, and if you find cylinder OD 95°, OS 35° you should take a second look.

FAR POINTS IN ASTIGMATISM

Retinoscopy in astigmatism often intimidates a novice, but with the simplified FP optics we have described this need not happen to you. Let's go back to the diagrammatic view of the emerging rays and start from scratch. Later in this chapter, you will get lots of practice to make sure that you grasp all of this.

Light leaving the retina is refracted differently by the principal corneal meridians. It is as though there were two eyes instead of one, each principal meridian acting like a separate eye. You can already

scope an eye with one principal meridian; all you need to do now is repeat the performance a second time on the same eye.

There are several phenomena you will observe with the retinoscope:

1. The eye will now have two reflexes, one in each principal meridian (Figure 7-2).

2. The speed, width, and brightness of the reflex will differ in the principal meridians.

3. The movement of the reflex will not be parallel to the movement of the face band (intercept) unless you are scoping along a principal meridian.

4. You cannot neutralize both meridians with a single lens, which is another way of saying there are two FPs.

Classification of Astigmatism

Let's look now at the five types of astigmatism described in Chapter 3. We will drop the superfluous degree mark (°) for the remainder of the chapter. I have placed the working lens in these diagrams to avoid confusing the relationship between

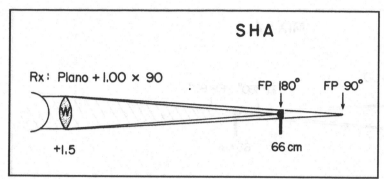

SHA

Rx: Plano + 1.00 × 90

FP 180°   FP 90°

W

+1.5

66 cm

Figure 7-3. Simple hyperopic astigmatism, uncorrected: one FP is where you are, the other is behind you. You would see NEUT in the 180 meridian and WITH in the 90 meridian (as in Figure 7-2).

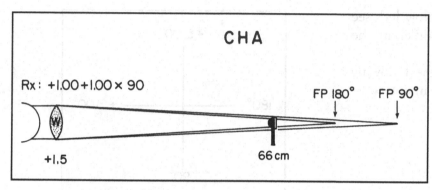

CHA

Rx: +1.00 +1.00 × 90

FP 180°   FP 90°

W

+1.5

66 cm

Figure 7-4. Compound hyperopic astigmatism, uncorrected: both FPs are behind you. Here you would see WITH in both meridians, but more WITH at 90.

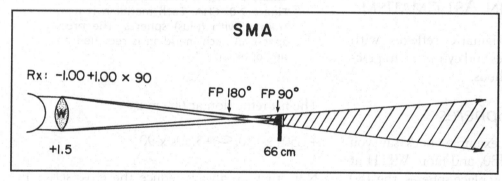

SMA

Rx: −1.00 +1.00 × 90

FP 180° FP 90°

W

+1.5

66 cm

Figure 7-5. Simple myopic astigmatism, uncorrected: one FP is in front of you. You would scope AGAINST at 180 and NEUT at 90.

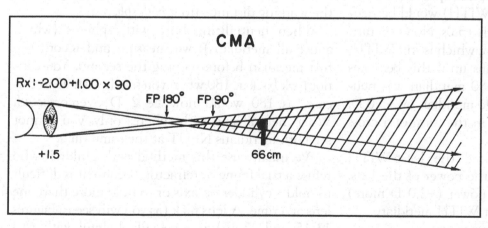

CMA

Rx: −2.00 +1.00 × 90

FP 180° FP 90°

W

+1.5

66 cm

Figure 7-6. Compound myopic astigmatism, uncorrected: both FPs are in front of you. Here you see AGAINST in both meridians, although there is more AGAINST at 180. However, degrees of AGAINST are hard to judge.

the FP and the neutralizing lenses. Rx refers to the correcting lenses *desired* (net) for neutralization (ignore this Rx for the moment as it may confuse you). Simply zoom through the diagrams (Figures 7-3 through 7-7), examining the FPs and reading the legends.

Figure 7-7. Mixed astigmatism: one FP is in front of you, the other behind you. You will see AGAINST in one meridian and WITH in the other.

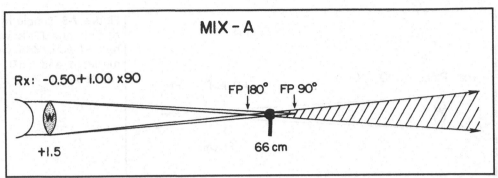

So much for the basic categories. Now let's see how we might handle reflexes that differ in the principal meridians.

Before proceeding, let's agree on the following abbreviations that are commonly used in optics:

s (sphere)
c (cylinder)
x (axis)
◯ (combined with)

NEUTRALIZATION IN ASTIGMATISM

We can neutralize astigmatic reflexes with spheres alone or with spheres and cylinders. In practice, you will use both methods.

Neutralizing With Spheres

We will start with an example. Let's say you scope and find WITH at 180, and more WITH at 90 (as in Figure 7-4). As you place spheres, the 180 meridian (having the lesser WITH) would be neutralized first, for example, with +3.0s. Now you turn your streak to the 90 meridian, which is still WITH, and you continue to add plus until this becomes NEUT at, say, +5.0s. The 180 meridian was neutralized by +3.0 D, and the 90 meridian by +5.0 D. You could record this value in the form of a cross (Figure 7-8).

Notice that we neutralized the least-WITH meridian first and recorded the power of the lens. Then we continued to add power (+2.0 D more) until we neutralized the most WITH meridian.

We could also record this *gross* as:

+3.0s x 180 ◯ +5.0s x 90

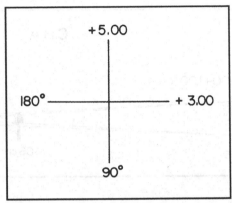

Figure 7-8. CHA. Each meridian is neutralized with (plus) spheres. The gross sphere in each meridian is recorded on an "optic cross."

The *net* refraction at 66 cm is:

+1.50s x 180 ◯ +3.50s x 90

Note that we always reduce the gross *sphere* by the working distance from *both spheres.*

When neutralizing only with spheres (which affect all meridians), we measure and record the first meridian before scoping the second. You cannot look back at 180 when you finish with 90 in this case, as 180 would now be 2 D overcorrected. When neutralizing with spheres only, you cannot see both meridians NEUT at the same time.

We usually use this method with children who refuse a trial frame or refractor, because it is difficult to hold a cylinder on axis or to hold more than one lens at a time. A lens rack (as you will see in Figures 13-15 and 13-18) is especially helpful with this technique in the office or when refracting under anesthesia.

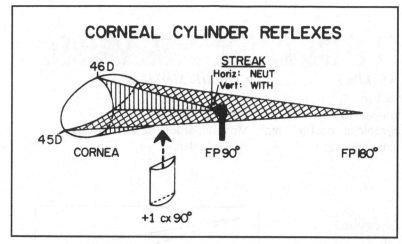

Figure 7-9. Effect of corneal cylinder on emerging rays. The 90 corneal meridian (+46 D) has FP at scope, so NEUT is seen when the streak is horizontal (testing the 90 meridian). The 180 corneal meridian has only +45 D, so it shows 1 D WITH when streak is vertical (testing the 180 meridian). Adding +1.0 x 90 will add power to 180, thus neutralizing the reflex seen at 90.

Neutralizing With Spheres and Cylinders

We could correct this same patient by neutralizing the first meridian with spheres, then adding cylinders to neutralize the second.

In our example, a +3.0s gave us NEUT at 180 and we call this the *spheric meridian.* Spheres apply power in all meridians, of course, so at 90 we would need +2.0 D more (it would still show 2 D WITH). Adding a +2.0c x 90 would neutralize this meridian without changing the reflex at 180 (because cylinders add power only to one meridian). We call this (residual WITH) meridian the *cylindric meridian* (what else?). So, both meridians would now be NEUT. Since you can *compare* meridians after neutralization by rotating your streak, this method is more accurate. The lenses before the eye would be:

+3.0s ⬯ +2.0c x 90

(The sphere is always written first.)

This is the gross refraction, mind you! Now we deduct the working distance from the sphere only, giving us:

+1.50s ⬯ +2.0c x 90.

We always write the sphere and cylinder in this order; thus, their symbols are superfluous (as is the ⬯), so in prescription shorthand we abbreviate this to:

+1.50 + 2.0 x 90.

Note that the total net *power,* scoped at the 90 meridian is actually +3.50 (+1.50s + 2.0c), the same as shown in the previous method.

Streak Meridian vs Corneal Meridian

At this point you might ask (everyone does!), "But the power of the cylinder axis 90 *acts* at 180! Since you saw more WITH at 90, wouldn't you place the axis at 180, in order to put the *power* at 90?" Good question.

The answer is that we are seeing retinoscopic reflexes, not corneal meridians. The WITH reflex we saw "at 90" is produced by the corneal *meridian* at 180. Your streak actually tests the power of the corneal meridian that it *sweeps across;* that is, the meridian perpendicular to the streak axis. For example, when we place the streak at 90 and move it side to side, we are actually examining the effect of the 180 meridian. So if we see WITH when the streak is *vertical* (sweeping the horizontal), the eye wants plus in the *horizontal* meridian. If we now place the correcting cylinder on the vertical (WITH) axis, its power is *applied* at 180, thus neutralizing the WITH reflex the 180 meridian had *produced* at 90. It is like a double negative, allowing you to forget the corneal meridian. You simply place *the axis of the plus cylinder over the axis of the WITH reflex.* Let's look at it (Figure 7-9).

The beauty of this plus cylinder system is that after neutralizing the spheric meridian, simply placing the cylinder axis on the *remaining-WITH* reflex axis will properly correct the corneal cylinder. The axis of the remaining WITH is the *plus cylinder* axis.

Table 7-1

	Spheric Meridian	Cylindric Meridian
	Characteristics of the Principal Meridians	
Power	Most refractive	Least refractive
FP	Closest to eye	Furthest from eye
Refraction	Least hyperopic or most myopic	Most hyperopic or least myopic
Neutralization	Plus or minus spheres	Plus cylinders

What we are actually doing in spherocylindric retinoscopy is first neutralizing the most refractive corneal meridian (the spheric) with spheres. Then we add plus to the least refractive meridian (the cylindric) alone, to make it equal the power of the spheric. At this point, both meridians are NEUT, and you have corrected the refractive error!

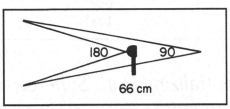

Figure 7-10. Simple hyperopic astigmatism: we see NEUT at 180, WITH at 90.

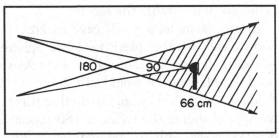

Figure 7-11. Simple myopic astigmatism: we see AGAINST at 180, NEUT at 90.

CLASSIFYING MERIDIANS

Before you become confused by the liberal use of synonyms in defining the principal meridians, let's tabulate the terms that are interchangeable (Table 7-1).

Now go back and look at Figures 7-3 through 7-7 again, this time comparing the location of the FPs with the Rx (the spheres and cylinders we will place to correct the refractive error).

In the illustrations, note that whatever the refraction, the FP *nearest* the eye is the *spheric* meridian; the *furthest* FP is the *cylindric* meridian. Once the spheric is NEUT, the cylindric meridian is *always* WITH, which makes it easy to manage with plus cylinders. (For simplicity, all these examples are "with the rule," so we'd place the cylindric axis at 90.)

Note how the FP in each illustration (Figures 7-3 through 7-7) would shift to 66 cm by the lens power applied in that meridian. In each case, would the Rx neutralize the situation? Do you understand how the FPs fulfill the characteristics of the principal meridians listed in Table 7-1?

ANALYZING THE APPROACH

Before looking at the reflexes, let's analyze what we will do when faced with differences in the meridians. In the series that follows, study the simplified diagram and decide how you would correct the situation, first with spheres, then with cylinders. Then, read the analysis that follows each example, making sure you understand the approach before proceeding.

Simple astigmatism. These really are simple, because one meridian is already NEUT. Let's examine both types of simple astigmatism diagrammatically, seeing ourselves amid the emerging cones of light (Figures 7-10 and 7-11).

In *simple hyperopic astigmatism* (SHA) (see Figure 7-10), which is the most common ametropia you will see, one meridian is NEUT and the other is WITH. Here we simply add a plus cylinder to the

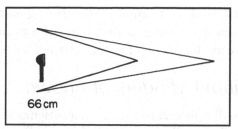

Figure 7-12. Compound hyperopic astigmatism: both meridians are WITH.

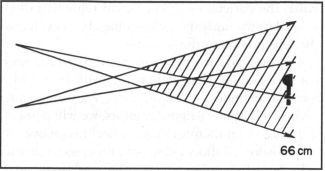

Figure 7-13. Compound myopic astigmatism: both meridians are AGAINST.

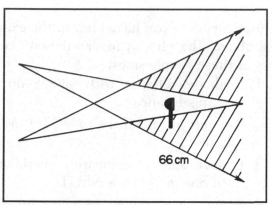

Figure 7-14. Mixed astigmatism: one meridian is WITH, the other AGAINST.

WITH meridian (90) until it too is NEUT. Nothing to it!

Simple myopic astigmatism (SMA) (see Figure 7-11) is a little trickier; there is NEUT in one meridian, but AGAINST in the other. In this case, you would add a *minus* sphere to push the myopic (180) meridian out, until the AGAINST becomes NEUT. Then, since the sphere will also have pushed out the previously NEUT (90) meridian, turning it to WITH, we will need a plus cylinder on this WITH (90) meridian to pull the FP back in to NEUT. Follow that?

Compound astigmatism. In these situations, neither meridian is NEUT, so the situation seems more difficult. But if you follow the rules, the three conditions are soon transformed into SHA. Remember to turn everything you see into WITH. Watch how that works (Figures 7-12 and 7-13).

Compound hyperopic astigmatism (CHA) (see Figure 7-12) is easy because both meridians are already WITH, although the amount differs. We add plus spheres until the least WITH (spheric) meridian is NEUT, then add our plus cylinder to neutralize the remaining WITH (cylindric) meridian. In practice, it is a simple matter to crank in plus spheres, rotating the streak, until one meridian first becomes NEUT, then simply add the plus cylinder to the opposite (remaining WITH) meridian.

In *compound myopic astigmatism* (see Figure 7-13) both meridians are AGAINST, but it is difficult to judge the value of the meridians when you see a double AGAINST reflex. We simply add minus spheres to push *both* FPs out beyond us, so we have friendly WITH in each meridian. Then proceed just as in CHA above: reduce the sphere until the first (most myopic) meridian is NEUT. Then add the cylinder to correct the remaining WITH reflex in the opposite (least myopic) meridian.

Mixed astigmatism (MIX-A). This is easy. We see AGAINST and WITH, so we simply add minus spheres until the AGAINST becomes WITH, then reduce the sphere until that meridian is NEUT. Then we use the cylinder to neutralize the remaining WITH, as always (Figure 7-14).

Now that we have mixed it up a little, let's review our principles again. We first neutralized the least hyperopic (or most myopic) meridian with spheres. The remaining meridian (the most hyperopic or least myopic) will always show WITH, which we adroitly handle with our plus cylinder. In other words, first neutralize the meridian with the FP closest to the eye with spheres, then close the astigmatic interval by applying the plus cylinder to the opposite (remaining-WITH) meridian, which has the FP furthest from the eye.

We have made no mention of the actual refractive error because it never concerns you during retinoscopy. You analyze the reflexes, take the appropriate steps to achieve NEUT in all meridians, correct this gross finding to net power and voila, the patient sees! The actual refraction often is not known until the lights come on and you read the lens powers in the refractor.

OK, enough theory; let's get to work. In the graduated exercises that follow, we will begin with medium cylinders of known axis. As we examine and correct these astigmatic errors, we will pause to illustrate the principles we have outlined above. As you develop confidence, we will progress to smaller cylinders, then unknown cylinders, and then (finally) unknown spherocylindric combinations.

Summary: As you have seen in the examples above, the plus cylinder method* consists of these simple steps:

1. Evaluate reflexes with sleeve up at working distance.
2. Convert all meridians to WITH, using spheres.
3. Reduce sphere, comparing meridians, until one meridian is NEUT.
4. Apply plus cylinder to neutralize the opposite meridian.
5. Move in and out a little, rotating streak, to compare meridians. Refine if necessary.
6. Check working distance. Result is the gross refraction.
7. Reduce sphere (only) by dioptric working distance to achieve net.

*For minus cylinder methods see p.92 and Chapter 10.

Astigmatic Reflexes

For these examples, we will avoid the working lens allowance by keeping your eye NEUT at the working distance. This will allow you to easily compare your neutralizing lenses with the prescription.

We will call this arrangement *emmetropia at the working distance* and will use it hereafter in astigmatism exercises. Set your eye at –1.5 on the corrected scale, *no working lens*. Check reflex at 66 cm, and adjust the sleeve if necessary. It is best here to stay

in a little WITH; it simplifies comparing meridians. Then tape the sleeve at that point. From now on, neutralizing lenses will produce the *net* correction.

Medium Cylinders of Known Axis

We will now create each of our astigmatic conditions and neutralize them step by step. Refer to the specific diagrams if you become disoriented. Be sure to use the correct phantom power, sign, and axis.

Exercise 14: Simple Hyperopic Astigmatism

Rx: Plano + 1.00 x 90 (see Figures 7-3 and 7-10) (Place phantom –1.0c x 90).

At 66 cm, sleeve up, streak horizontal (180), you have NEUT.[†] Rotate the streak to 90 meridian, to see WITH. OK? It is apparent that 180 is the spheric meridian and 90 is the meridian of the plus cylinder (cylindric). Let's look at it another way:

Move in about 20 cm (8 inches) and rotate streak between 90 and 180. Note the difference in width, speed, and brightness. 180 is wider and slower, thus closer to NEUT. 90 is narrower and faster, thus further from NEUT. Since 180 has the *least* WITH, it is the spheric meridian; the 90 meridian has the *most* WITH, so it is the *cylindric* meridian.

Now ease back slowly to 66 cm, rotating the streak to compare meridians and see that 180 fills first. Since this spheric meridian is NEUT at working distance, it needs no further attention. The cylindric axis still shows WITH.

Add +0.50c x 90. Compare meridians. Is 90 NEUT yet?

Remove the last lens and replace it with +1.0c x 90. Compare meridians. Move back and forth to see that both meridians are NEUT at about the same distance.

Compare correcting lens with Rx above (ignore phantom). Easy, isn't it?

Exercise 15: Compound Hyperopic Astigmatism

Rx: +1.00 + 1.00 x 90 (see Figures 7-4 and 7-12) (Place phantom –1.0s, then –1.0c x 90).

[†]*Note that the phantom cylinder axis is 90, while exerting its power at 180 does not affect what you see with the streak at 180. That is because power in the 180 meridian is seen when the streak is at 90. Thus the effect of a cylinder is on its axis. Refer back to Figure 7-9 if this is not clear.*

Compare meridians: is there *less* WITH at 180? Since both meridians are WITH, you will add plus spheres until the first (or least) WITH is NEUT, then plus cylinders will neutralize the opposite meridian.

Neutralize the spheric meridian in +0.50 D steps. Is it more or less NEUT at +1.0s?

Now neutralize the cylindric meridian in +0.50 D steps (If you have run out of cells, just hold up the cylinder close to the stack. Watch the axis; it must be exact for neutralization). Whenever the fourth place in the stack is the plus cylinder, you may find it slightly overcorrects the minus cylinder phantom; plus lenses get stronger with increased VD.

Compare meridians at working distance. Your correcting lenses should equal the Rx above (ignoring phantoms).

In the following exercises, remember that you must *first* deal with AGAINST. Since it is too confusing to approach NEUT from the AGAINST direction, always overcorrect it to WITH, then reduce power to neutralize.

Exercise 16: Simple Myopic Astigmatism

Rx: −1.00 + 1.00 x 90 (see Figures 7-5 and 7-11) (Place phantom + 1.0c x 180; note sign and axis).

Compare meridians. Do you see NEUT at 90? (Lean in a little to confirm.) Is there AGAINST at 180? This is the spheric meridian (FP closest to the eye), so we start here.

With streak at 180, add −0.50s. Is it less AGAINST? (Hard to tell!)

Replace last lens with −1.0s. 180 should be NEUT now.

Check the cylindric meridian. What happened to the previous NEUT? Is it now WITH?

Neutralize 90 with cylinders in 0.50 D steps. When both meridians are NEUT, compare correcting lenses with Rx above (ignore phantom). You should be right on.

Exercise 17: Compound Myopic Astigmatism

Rx: −2.00 + 1.00 x 180 (see Figures 7-6 and 7-13) (Place phantom +2.0s, and −1.0c x 180).

Compare meridians. Are both AGAINST? Is there less AGAINST at 180? Which is the spheric meridian? (Tough question?)

Degrees of AGAINST are difficult. Try this: zoom in with the sleeve up until both are WITH, then ease back, comparing meridians, until the first is NEUT. The meridian with the FP closest to the eye is *always* the spheric. The opposite meridian will still show WITH, so it is the cylindric. Smooth move!

Now, go back to 66 cm, and neutralize the spheric meridian you have found. Plus or minus spheres? (If uncertain of your endpoint, overcorrect a little to WITH, then reduce sphere.)

While neutralizing 90, note that 180 is also changing. When the spheric meridian is NEUT, what has happened to the cylindric? Why?

How will you now approach 180? Neutralize cylindric in +0.50 D steps. Keep cylinder on axis.

When 180 is NEUT, recheck 90. Compare with Rx. Note that this is a case of "*against* the rule" astigmatism (the plus cylinder axis is horizontal).

Exercise 18: Mixed Astigmatism

Rx: −0.50 + 1.00 x 45 (see Figures 7-7 and 7-14) (Place phantom +0.50s and −1.0c x 45).

At 66 cm, sleeve up, rotate streak and survey reflex. Be sure to wiggle the scope perpendicular to the streak axis. Interesting? What do you see and where? Do not read further until you try to sort this one out.

One meridian is AGAINST and the other is WITH. We wish to neutralize the spheric meridian first, right? Which is it?

How do we locate the spheric "axis"? One way is to place the streak *perpendicular* to the WITH (cylindric) band at 45. We expect the principal meridians to be 90° apart. Use the more accurate way: with the sleeve up, move in until all meridians are WITH. Then slowly recede, rotating streak (maintain optical alignment). You will see that 135 fills first; that makes it the spheric (the FP closest to the eye, right?). At that point 45 has lots of WITH, so it is clearly the cylindric. Marvelous! Moving in is a very helpful maneuver.

So, we neutralize the spheric first. Move back to 66 cm, streak at 135, and neutralize that meridian. With what? Be sure to wiggle perpendicular to *streak* axis. And maintain alignment, watching the pupil center. You should find NEUT with –0.50s. OK?

Neutralize the cylindric meridian, starting with +0.50c. If you have to hold up the correcting cylinder, note that you must be *exactly* on axis to neutralize. +1.0c x 45 should do it, or slightly overcorrect (VD, you know.).

Compare with prescription. This is a case of *oblique* astigmatism.

If you are feeling good about these five exercises, give yourself a few strokes. You have confronted all combinations of reflexes and neutralized them. You have moved in to compare meridians, located the principal meridians at various axes, and know which to approach first.

DETECTING SMALLER CYLINDERS

It should now be obvious that anyone can see a 1 D cylinder. Let's develop a little finesse, now, in detecting smaller cylinders. We will start with a neutrality background to make the cylinder easy to locate and measure.

Recheck emmetropia at working distance with no working lens.

Exercise 19

With-the-rule 0.75 D c:
(Place phantom –0.75c x 90)

Rotate streak to compare meridians. The cylinder is obvious, right?

Neutralize cylinder in +0.25 steps; practice comparing meridians as you go. Watch optical alignment.

Exercise 20

Against-the-rule 0.50 D c:
(Place phantom –0.50c x 180)

This time, use the *left* eye, left hand, and both eyes open.

Compare meridians. Is a 0.50 cylinder easy to find?

Place +0.25c x 180. Compare meridians. There is still 0.25 D of WITH. Could you miss that? Does it help to move in when comparing?

Exercise 21

Oblique 0.25 D c:
(Place phantom –0.25c x 45)

Rotate the streak, comparing meridians. Could you miss a 0.25 D cylinder if you only checked 90 and 180? A useful maneuver here is to move back beyond working distance; all meridians show AGAINST except 45, revealing the cylinder location.

Exercise 22

Unknown 0.25 D c:
(Have a helper rotate the same phantom to *any* axis.)

Compare meridians. Can you find the cylinder?

Repeat this several times, while rotating axes and alternating right and left eyes. When one meridian is *first* made NEUT, even a 0.25 D cylinder is easy to find, if you look. Just be sure not to "overfill" the NEUT meridian (ie, keep a little WITH in the pupil center).

Exercise 23

Mini 0.12 D c:
(Place phantom –0.12c x 100)
Compare meridians. Can you see it?
Rotate to some oblique axis. Can you find it? Surprised?

Review of Plus Cylinder Method

Before we let you loose on unknown astigmatic conditions, let's quickly review just what you are doing when you approach meridians with differing reflexes.

It should be clear from the introductory exercises that we can reduce the five types of astigmatism to three situations: 1) *both* reflexes are WITH, 2) *one* reflex is WITH, or 3) *neither* reflex is WITH.

> **From this, we can simplify the plus cylinder approach:**
> 1. Both reflexes are WITH (CHA): Add plus spheres until the first (spheric) meridian is NEUT. Then add plus cylinders to the remaining WITH (cylindric) meridian.
> 2. One reflect is WITH (SHA, MIX-A): Move in until both are WITH, then ease back, comparing meridians until the first (spheric) is NEUT; shift this FP to 66 cm with minus spheres. Correct remaining WITH using plus cylinders.
> 3. Neither reflex is WITH (CMA, SMA): Proceed exactly as in (2), above.

Once you get down to the fundamentals, it is surprising how little you need to know. In fact, the method can be simplified still further, to only two situations: 1) both reflexes *are* WITH, or 2) *they are not.*

- *First situation*: if both reflexes are WITH, you will proceed as in number 1.
- *Second situation*: if both reflexes are not WITH, you will proceed as in 2.

So much for review; now you are on your own.

UNKNOWN SPHERES WITH SMALL CYLINDERS

In the series that follows, we will use an *unknown* sphere, with progressively smaller cylinders of knows axis. You will have to first *create* your own neutral background (spheric meridian) to determine the amount of cylinder. Follow each exercise carefully.

If you have a *five* cell schematic eye, it is best to continue using phantom *spheres* to create a verifiable refractive error. Keep your eye set for *emmetropia* at working distance.

If you have a *three* cell model, and are annoyed by having to hold up the fourth lens, you may use the dioptric *scale* to create the spherical error. This is less accurate for sphere, but the cylinder will be true, since the astigmatism is created by a phantom.

Remember to deduct 1.5 D from the gross to calculate the net refraction, since we have abandoned the working lens.

Exercise 24

Unknown, with the rule (1.0 D c):
Have your partner or helper create low sphere error (up to ±2 D) by whichever method you have chosen for your model eye. Add phantom −1.0c x 90.

Compare meridians, and decide what you have. Check the proper category, as described earlier, to review your approach.

Neutralize the *spheric* meridian (closest FP, least WITH, or most AGAINST).

Neutralize the *cylindric* meridian, starting with +0.50c, then in +0.25c steps.

Compare meridians, checking optical alignment and working distance.

Record correcting lenses. Compare with phantom (or with scale on eye, minus working distance power, if you have chosen that method). Are you close?

Exercise 25

Unknown, against the rule (0.50 D c):
(Have partner create low sphere error, then add −0.50c x 180)

This time, use your *left* eye, holding the scope in your left hand. Keep both eyes open.

Compare meridians. What do you see? What will you do? Do it.

Neutralize as above, comparing your correction with the refractive error. Getting better? OK, you may go back to your right eye.

Exercise 26

Unknown, oblique (0.25 D c):
(Create low sphere error, adding −0.25c x 60)

Compare meridians as before. It is easy to fall into the trap of concentrating on 90/180, and in haste you can miss a small cylinder.

Unknown Spherocylinder Combinations

Now you are ready to really try your wings.

Exercise 27: Double Unknown

Have your helper create a low (±2 D) sphere error, then place –0.50c phantom on *any* axis.

Try this one with your *left* eye.

Repeat several times with different sphere errors and phantom cylinder axes.

Exercise 28: Triple Unknown

Create low sphere error, then place any low cylinder (0.75c or less) on any axis.

Go for it!

Well, you have come a long way in this chapter, and at this point you know as much as many practitioners ever know about retinoscopy. In the next chapter, we will get into some special techniques for determining and refining cylinder axis and power.

8

REFINING THE CYLINDER

"Treat nature in terms of the cylinder, the sphere, the cone, all in perspective."

Paul Cezanne

Now that you are acquainted with retinoscopy in astigmatism, we will proceed with some ancillary techniques for determining and refining the axis and power of the cylinder. Much of this will seem repetitious, but the practice will prove useful later on.

ESTIMATING CYLINDER AXIS

Four phenomena help in finding the axis: *break*, *width*, *intensity*, and *skew*. You have *seen* all of these already, but have not really *observed* them. All four result from the axis reflexes and oblique motion you observe when the streak is not on the cylinder meridian. You can study these phenomena best when the astigmatic reflex is *enhanced*, so let's review enhancement again.

Enhancement

When we adjust the sleeve height of the retinoscope to produce the brightest, narrowest fundus reflex, we call this the position of *enhancement*. You may recall that we touched on this earlier, in Chapter 6. We can see the enhanced astigmatic reflex best against a background of neutrality (Figure 8-1).

We see small cylinders best with the plane mirror (ie, when the sleeve is up). Larger cylinders can be enhanced by lowering the sleeve. With enhancement, the astigmatic band becomes brighter, sharper, narrower, and more distinct (Figure 8-2).

Recall that the intercept is the streak image on the *surface* of the eye. In Figure 8-2, you can see that if the reflex is narrowest when the intercept is *wide* (ie, in the sleeve up position), the cylinder power is low. If the retinal reflex is narrowest when the intercept is *narrow* (ie, with the sleeve lowered), the cylinder power is high. We are changing the vergence of the beam from diverging rays (sleeve up), to converging rays, which focus on the schematic eye (when the sleeve is at midpoint). Because instruments vary, it is not the sleeve height, but the *width of the intercept* when the reflex is enhanced that makes this technique reliable. We cannot enhance cylinders greater than 5 D by lowering the sleeve beyond the midpoint; converging the beam any further produces reversal of the retinal reflex and blurring (broadening) of the intercept (but you will seldom see cylinder powers higher than 5 D).

Let's look at two examples to illustrate this technique.

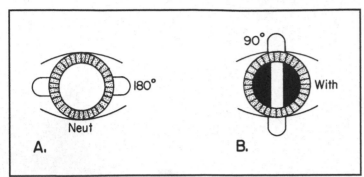

Figure 8-1. Neutral meridian. We create a neutral spheric meridian in order to see the cylindric reflex most clearly. The NEUT reflex at 180 (A) clearly reveals the WITH at 90 (B). We would now lower the sleeve in this cylindric meridian to try enhancing the reflex.

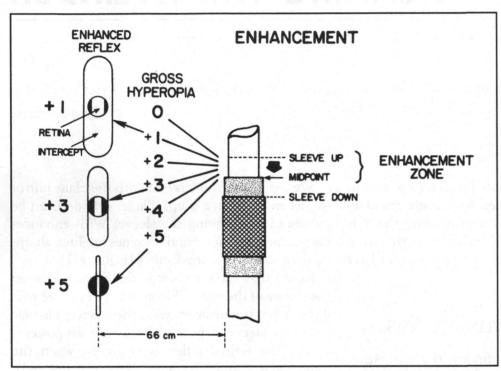

Figure 8-2. Enhancement. At working distance, lower the sleeve to produce the narrowest (enhanced) retinal reflex. The enhancement zone is between sleeve up and about halfway down (midpoint). Judge the approximate power of the cylinder by the width of the intercept when the retinal reflex is enhanced.

Exercise 29: Enhancement, Large Cylinder

Your schematic eye should be set for emmetropia at working distance (approximately –1.5 on your corrected scale, no working lens).

Check NEUT at 66 cm and refine if necessary. Tape the sleeve at this position. Place a phantom –2.0c x 85.

With the sleeve up, rotate your streak to compare meridians. The WITH reflex clearly reveals the approximate cylinder axis.

Lower the sleeve, watching the retinal cylinder reflex. You will see that it can be enhanced. There is a point where it is brightest, sharpest, narrowest, and most distinct. Note the sleeve height and width

of the intercept at this point. This *sleeve* height (which will vary among instruments) is the approximate position for enhancing 2 D of astigmatism. The *intercept* width is the precise indication of a 2 D cylinder. If you lower the sleeve further, the reflex will broaden again.

Exercise 30: Enhancement, Small Cylinder

Remove the lens and replace it with a phantom –0.50c x 105. Use your left eye.

Compare meridians with the sleeve up. You can see the WITH band at the approximate cylindric axis.

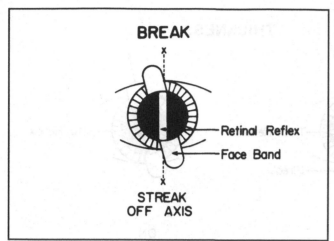

BREAK

Retinal Reflex

Face Band

STREAK OFF AXIS

Figure 8-3. Break. The line between the streak in the pupil and outside the pupil is broken when the streak is off the correct axis.

Lower the sleeve while watching the reflex. Note that it does not become narrower and brighter. In fact, it becomes broader and duller! Small cylinders cannot be enhanced by lowering the sleeve.

Thus, lowering the sleeve enhances a large cylinder; sleeve up "enhances" a small cylinder. The farther down the sleeve you see enhancement, the larger the cylinder. (This technique is also useful for estimating the power of the cylinder, so we will see it again.) Because most astigmatism is small and cannot be enhanced, many practitioners forget to lower the sleeve when they encounter medium and higher cylinders.

Now let's use enhancement against the neutral meridian to observe the four axis phenomena in detail. Because these exercises involve comparison of the reflex and intercept, be sure to darken the room so you can see the intercept clearly.

Recheck NEUT at 66 cm. Place a phantom −2.00c x 90, but turn the lens around so you cannot see the score mark from the front. With sleeve up, the spheric meridian is NEUT and the cylindric meridian is WITH.

Enhance the cylindric reflex. As you read the following, confirm these observations with the reflex enhanced.

Exercise 31: Break Phenomenon

We observe break when the streak is off-axis. When the intercept (face band) and the streak reflex are not parallel, they form a broken line (Figure 8-3), which you can see simply by rotating the streak to either side of the astigmatic reflex.

The break disappears when the intercept and reflex are parallel (ie, when the streak is on the axis). We place the correcting cylinder on this unbroken line. Try it. Keep your sleeve at the position of enhancement and rotate the streak to about 15° on either side of the axis (ie, from 75 to 115). Note that break is most marked at the extremes of this arc and decreases as you approach the axis. There is no break at 90, so this will be the axis for your correcting cylinder. Do not forget to judge break when the reflex is enhanced. Repeating these observations with the sleeve up should convince you that the exact axis is not nearly so clear without enhancement.

Observing break proves essential in locating large cylinders (try it within a phantom −5.0c), but it proves no help in dealing with astigmatism under 1.0 D.

Exercise 32: Thickness Phenomenon

When you rotate the streak to either side of the correct axis, the *thickness* (or width) of the reflex varies. The reflex appears narrowest when the streak aligns with the axis, and wider when it is off alignment.

Turn the −2.0c phantom to axis 75.

Enhance the reflex. Rotate the streak to 15° on either side of the cylindric meridian (ie, from 60 to 90) observing how the reflex varies in width (Figure 8-4).

Now turn the phantom to a random meridian and repeat these rotations. Use your left eye to observe variations in width of the reflex. When the reflex is narrowest, compare your axis with the score mark on the phantom.

Exercise 33: Intensity Phenomenon

The *intensity* of the reflex changes slightly as we rotate the streak about the cylindric meridian. The reflex is brightest when the streak is on the correct axis.

This observation is subtle and useful only in small cylinders that you cannot enhance (with large cylinders, the enhanced reflex is already bright).

Figure 8-4. Thickness. We locate the axis where the retinal reflex is the thinnest.

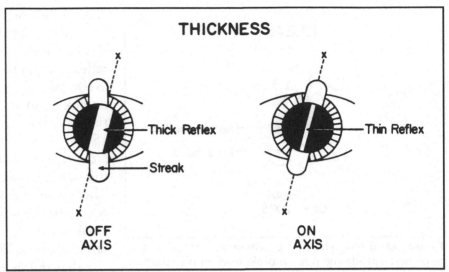

THICKNESS

Thick Reflex

Streak

OFF AXIS

Thin Reflex

ON AXIS

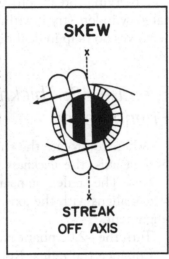

SKEW

STREAK OFF AXIS

Figure 8-5. Skew (oblique motion). The arrows indicating movement of the reflex and intercept are not parallel. The reflex and intercept do not move in the same direction, but are skewed when the streak is off-axis.

Replace your phantom with a –0.25c x 105. Observe that you cannot enhance small cylinders by lowering the sleeve. Where will you place the sleeve height to achieve the narrowest reflex?

Rotate the streak about the axis and note that the reflex is slightly duller at 75 and 135, and somewhat brighter at 105 (this takes less imagination with real eyes, where the reflex is dimmer). While this phenomenon may not seem very useful, with small cylinders you sometimes need all the help you can get.

Exercise 34: Skew Phenomenon

We use *skew* (sometimes called oblique motion) to refine more precisely the axis in small cylinders. This is the only one of these four phenomena in which we do not rotate the streak. We wiggle the streak (perpendicular to its axis, as always) in a zone of about 30° to either side of the apparent axis, while comparing the *motion* of the reflex with that of the intercept.

The reflex moves *parallel* to the intercept when the streak is on the axis. When the streak is off the axis, the reflex and intercept move in different directions; that is, their motion is skewed (Figure 8-5).

Replace the lens with a phantom –0.50c x 90, turned around so you cannot see the axis mark. Check NEUT at 180.

Place the streak at about 60 and watch the *reflex* while wiggling the streak perpendicular to its axis. Repeat this at 120. The intercept and reflex are not moving parallel. You can also see this oblique motion with the streak 15° off-axis; that is, at 75 and 105. Try it.

Do you agree that the movements are skewed in all but 90 meridian?

Rotate the phantom to some unknown meridian. Locate the axis using skew.

Now, lower your sleeve (about halfway) until the *intercept* is enhanced on the face of the model eye. Use this sharp line to pinpoint your axis, then compare this with the hidden axis of your phantom. Are you close?

Let's pause a moment to look at this "enhancement of the intercept" more closely; it will come in handy. When you have decided on the cylindric axis, lower your sleeve further to enhance the inter-

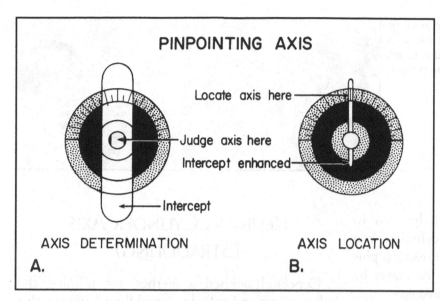

PINPOINTING AXIS

Locate axis here

Judge axis here

Intercept enhanced

Intercept

AXIS DETERMINATION
A.

AXIS LOCATION
B.

Figure 8-6. Locating axis on the protractor. First determine the astigmatic axis (A). Then lower the sleeve to enhance the intercept until the filament is seen as a fine line pinpointing the axis (B).

cept, being careful not to rotate the streak off your chosen axis (to ignore the reflex in the pupil, it helps to lower the scope from your eye and look over it). The enhanced intercept line will illuminate the degree mark on the protractor of the schematic eye or refractor; this is the line you will choose for the axis of your correcting cylinder (Figure 8-6).

When you are locating the axis, all four of these phenomena contribute to your decision. Break and thickness are most helpful with higher cylinders, and intensity and skew are most useful with low cylinders. As you have seen, it is natural to make use of several phenomena simultaneously. Ultimately, you will determine the axis in an almost completely unconscious process, using all of these clues.

ESTIMATING CYLINDER POWER

As you know, the wider the pupillary reflex band, the closer your meridian is to neutrality. Once the spheric meridian is NEUT, the width of the astigmatic reflex indicates the *power* of the cylinder. As a rule, the thinner the reflex in the cylindric meridian, the greater the astigmatism. If the streak is wide, you are nearer NEUT, so of course there is less astigmatism.

In low astigmatism, which you cannot enhance, the width of the pupil *reflex* gives the best estimate of cylinder power. In higher astigmatism, in which

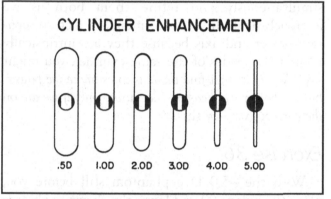

CYLINDER ENHANCEMENT

.5D   1.0D   2.0D   3.0D   4.0D   5.0D

Figure 8-7. Width of the intercept and reflex in various powers of WITH motion (reprinted from Copeland JC. *Streak Retinoscopy*. Chicago, Ill: Stereo Optical Company, Inc; 1967:15. Courtesy of Stereo Optical Co Inc.).

the *intercept* and reflex narrow increasingly as you enhance larger cylinders, the intercept gives us the most accurate indication of power. In Figure 8-7, the sleeve is lowered to the position of maximum enhancement of the pupillary reflex. Note the increasing narrowness of the reflex and the intercept in the higher cylinder powers. (We illustrated this technique in Figure 8-2.)

Exercise 35

Get phantom cylinders of –1.0, –3.0, and –5.0 D. Observe each in turn, at random axes.

Lower your sleeve to enhance the reflex and compare the width of the reflex and the intercept. Are your observations similar to those in the figure?

Figure 8-8. Maintaining fixation. An assortment of colorful, noisy toys, and talent for barnyard sounds and facial contortions help keep the fundus reflex in view. A strong mother helps to keep the patient still.

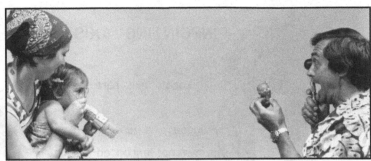

Do you see how enhancement helps you to quickly estimate the power of the cylinder? You would now place the approximate correcting plus cylinder, and then proceed to refine the power by neutralization technique with the sleeve up.

In practice, we estimate cylinder power and axis simultaneously and refine them both as we approach neutrality. It is artificial, in fact, to separate power and axis because they are intrinsically related (two sides of the same cylinder, you might say). *We must first find the axis to estimate the power, but the power we measure is accurate only if we are on the correct axis.* Try this:

Exercise 36

With the –5.0 D c phantom still before you, place the axis at 90 and lower the sleeve to observe the enhanced reflex when you are on the axis. Now turn the streak to 120 and raise the sleeve to the top. Slowly lower the sleeve again to "enhance" this off-axis reflex. When the reflex is the thinnest, we are seeing the cylinder power 30° off the axis. Now, keeping sleeve height the same, rotate the streak back to 90. From here you can lower the sleeve *further* to enhance; thus, there is more power in this (axis) meridian. This means that the power of the cylinder appears reduced when you are off the cylindric axis (ie, you will underestimate the power of the cylinder if your axis is incorrect).

But never underestimate the power of a child to look anywhere *but* in the right direction. This child's (Figure 8-8) last feeding was withheld, so she is pacified by the overdue bottle. Cycloplegic drops control her accommodation (p. 117), so fixation on near targets is acceptable.

Well, so much for estimating the axis and power. Now let's look at how to refine these estimations.

REFINING CYLINDER AXIS (STRADDLING)

Copeland devised a method for refining the cylinder *axis* and called it "straddling." We use this technique with the approximate correcting cylinder in place. Try it for yourself.

Exercise 37: Straddling

Check emmetropia at working distance (NEUT at working distance without working lens).

Place phantom –2.0c x 90 (this represents the cylindric axis of the eye).

Place a +2.0c x 80. This is your correcting cylinder (sometimes called the glass cylinder), with an axis error of 10° (Figure 8-9).

Straddling meridians are at 45° off to either side of the glass cylinder. We compare them with the sleeve up.

Now move in close to the model eye until you see a narrow reflex in each of the straddling meridians; that is, at about 35 and 125.

Move back about 10 cm, and rotate your streak to compare the straddling meridians. Recede further, and compare them again (sleeve up!). Repeat this until one of the meridians begins to widen or neutralize before the other. Is it the meridian at 35 or 125? The reflex in the straddling meridians is not equal at the same distance, so there is an *axis error*.

We call the persisting *narrow* reflex the "guide" line. As you recede and compare meridians, the 125 meridian remains narrow while 35 broadens, so this narrow line becomes your *guide*.

To correct this axis error, we turn our plus cylinder axis *toward* the guide. Rotate the correcting cylinder axis to 85, and move in again to compare the straddling meridians 45° to each side of the new glass axis. Is there a guide indicating axis error?

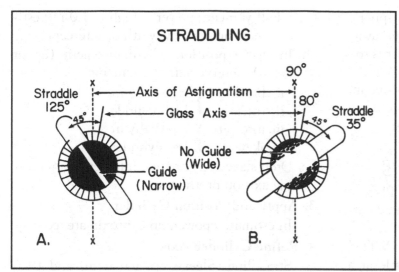

STRADDLING

Figure 8-9. Straddling. The straddling meridians are 45° off the glass axis, at roughly 35 and 125. As you move back from the eye while comparing meridians, the reflex at 125 remains narrow (A) at the same distance that the reflex at 35 has become wide (B). This dissimilarity indicates axis error; the narrow reflex (A) is the guide toward which we must turn the glass axis.

Move the cylinder axis 2° toward the guide and repeat straddling. As you reduce the angle of error, the guide loses its sharpness. When there is no axis error, there is no guide and straddling meridians will be similar as you move back to working distance.

Try this exercise with other cylinder pairs: first, −3.0/+3.0, then, −1.0/+1.0. Let someone place the phantom axis on a random meridian, with the correcting cylinder about 10° off-axis; conceal the axes of both lenses.

This is excellent practice. You can see that straddling is very accurate in high astigmatism, less helpful in low cylinders. Copeland even used this technique to detect tiny errors in alignment between trial cylinder lenses and the axis marks on their handles! Straddling helps us most in high astigmatism, which is the very situation that demands accurate placement of the correcting cylinder. You will find straddling especially valuable with children, who cannot subjectively refine the axis by cross cylinder testing (see Chapter 13).

REFINING CYLINDER POWER

"You can accurately locate the cylinder axis with an incorrect cylinder power," Copeland said, "but you cannot determine the correct cylinder power with an incorrect axis." While this principle may seem confusing, it rests firmly on logic and is the reason we *always refine the axis of the cylinder before refining the power.*

There is nothing new here. Now that we have refined the axis, we refine cylinder *power* by comparing the reflexes in the principal meridians at working distance. Since this technique is already familiar to you, I would like to suggest now that you move in to compare these meridians at a point *closer* than the working distance. This method is more accurate (and usually quicker) than those you have used because you can best detect small differences in the meridians by comparing the locations of their FPs (see Figure 6-3). To use this method with minus cylinders, refer to page 92.

We begin with the spheric meridian neutralized and our estimated correcting cylinder on the refined axis.

Exercise 38: Cylinder Too Weak

Check emmetropia at working distance. Place phantom −1.0c x 90, with +0.75c x 90 (your estimated correcting cylinder) right over it.

Move in with your sleeve up until you see a good, narrow WITH band in both meridians.

Now recede, rotating the streak to compare meridians. Note that the reflexes do not broaden or fill equally. That is, at some distance the reflex in one meridian will begin to broaden before the other; their FPs are not the same distance from the eye. Which meridian begins to fill first? Is this the spheric meridian? This illustrates a retinoscopy maxim: *"If the spheric fills first, the cylinder is too weak."*

This means that if the reflex in the spheric meridian broadens or fills first as you move away from the eye, the power of your plus cylinder is too low.

Add a +0.25c x 90 to the other lenses. Move in, then recede, comparing meridians as before; note that the reflexes broaden symmetrically now.

Exercise 39: Cylinder Too Strong

Keep the same –1.0 phantom c x 90. Place a +1.25c x 90 over it, to serve as your estimated correcting cylinder. Use your left eye this time.

Move in close, sleeve up, to see a narrow WITH band in both meridians. Now recede a little at a time, comparing meridians as before.

Which meridian fills first, spheric or cylindric?

Time for another maxim: *"If the cylindric fills first, the cylinder is too strong."*

This means that your plus cylinder has too much power.

Place a correcting –0.25c x 90 over these lenses, move in, then move back as before. Note the symmetrical filling of the principal meridians. Are both meridians NEUT at working distance?

SUMMARY

Now it is time to summarize all the principles and techniques we have learned thus far. We will follow an ordered progression that carries you from unknown ametropia to NEUT in all meridians. These we call the six steps of neutralization.

Six Steps of Neutralization

1. Apply Sphere
   a. Sleeve up, survey reflex (you may wish to move in at first to find WITH, thus locating the FPs).
   b. Apply spheres to get WITH in all meridians at working distance.
   c. Neutralize spheric (weakest or least WITH) meridian by adding plus (or reducing minus).

2. Estimate Cylinder Power and Axis
   a. In remaining WITH meridian, drop sleeve to attempt enhancement:
      i. If you cannot, power is low (<1.0 D).

      ii. If you can, power is high (>1.0 D); estimate amount by width of intercept.
   b. In sleeve position of enhancement (up or down), observe axis phenomena:
      i. break $\Big\}$ especially in
      ii. thickness $\Big\}$ high cylinders
      iii. intensity $\Big\}$ especially in
      iv. skew $\Big\}$ low cylinders
   c. Drop sleeve to enhance intercept, pinpointing axis on protractor.

3. Apply and Position Cylinder
   In estimated power, on approximate axis.

4. Refine Cylinder Axis
   Straddling. Sleeve up, move in, and then recede in straddling meridians, following the guideline.

5. Refine Cylinder Power
   Sleeve up, move in, and then recede, comparing principle meridians. Adjust plus cylinder power until meridians fill equally at the same distance.

6. Refine Sphere
   Check distance, adjusting the sphere (if necessary) to bring NEUT to 66 cm.

You should proceed this way in every case until the steps become a habit; only then are you allowed to take shortcuts.

Practice Exercises

Apply the preceding steps *one at a time* to the two following situations:

Exercise 40

Have a partner set the eye for myopic refractive error, about –2.0 or –2.5.

Place a –1.00 cylinder axis 80 or 100.

Neutralize this, step-by-step. When done, record your "gross" findings, subtract working distance to get "net," and compare with eye. Are you close? Is cylinder closer than sphere?

Exercise 41

Have a partner set the eye for plano and place a –0.50 cylinder axis at 10 or 170. Neutralize and compare as above.

Technique Exercises

Set the eye at NEUT at 66 cm, no working lens.

Exercise 42

Place –0.50c x 45.

Make a standard approach, scanning the 90 and 180 meridians. Is it quickly apparent that "something is amiss" at 90/180? Find NEUT axis. Find the astigmatic axis. Neutralize it.

Exercise 43

Replace cylinder with –0.25c x 90.

Compare principal meridians, convincing yourself there is astigmatism. Place correcting +0.25c x 85, and do axis checks. Do they guide you to the correct axis?

Exercise 44

Unknown: axis determination.

Replace with –1.00 cylinder and have your partner rotate to any axis. You determine axis.

Place +1.00 correcting cylinder over found axis. Refine cylinder axis by *straddling* technique. Compare meridians. All should be NEUT now.

Exercise 45

Unknown: axis determination.

Replace with –0.50 cylinder, have your partner rotate. Determine axis.

Place only +0.25 cylinder over found axis. Refine axis by straddling. Refine power now.

Exercise 46

Unknown: axis determination.

Replace with –0.25 cylinder. Have your partner rotate. Determine axis. Correct axis and power. If within 10°, you win!

Practice with unknown aspheric ametropias. Have your helper adjust your schematic eye to any spherical error, and then add any phantom minus cylinder at random with the axis mark concealed.

Follow each of the steps in turn, until you have NEUT in all meridians. Then record the total power of the lenses before the eye (except phantom cylinder) as your gross; subtract working distance to get net. Compare your *sphere* with the corrected scale on your schematic eye and your *cylinder* with the power and axis of the phantom. Are you close? You should be consistently within 0.25 D of sphere and cylinder if you have accurately calibrated your training eye. If it is not accurate, and you have a five-cell model, set it for emmetropia at working distance and use a phantom sphere.

Change the sphere error, choose a new phantom cylinder on a random axis, and repeat this with your left eye.

Go over these steps repeatedly until you are familiar with the sequence and confident of your work.

Congratulations! You are becoming an expert!

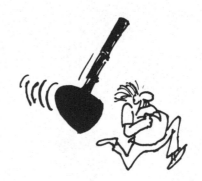

9

ESTIMATING TECHNIQUES AND MORE

"I have developed a method of refracting a deaf,
or dumb person in a few minutes—without lenses!"

Jack C. Copeland (at age 25)

If you feel fairly confident of your accomplishments so far, be assured that you do not have to learn any more techniques to become a good retinoscopist. You need only transfer your skills from the schematic eye to real people, then perfect the art of retinoscopy by repetition and self-analysis. There are some additional methods, collectively called "estimating techniques" that prove helpful in your retinoscopy repertoire. In this chapter, we will briefly discuss these techniques and some other subjects that do not naturally fit anywhere else.

ESTIMATING WITHOUT LENSES

When refractionists did all retinoscopy with trial frames (see Figure 13-7), the ability to make a preliminary estimate of the ametropia *without lenses* had great value, mainly because it took so much time to change the lenses when neutralizing. Copeland, for example, could determine a refractive error of +10.0 + 3.0 x 122 in seconds *without lenses*, using the techniques we will study. While employed in his youth by a department store to refract immigrants for a few cents per head, he perfected the art as a matter of necessity. Since he could not easily communicate with his patients, and success depended on high volume (with accuracy), Copeland developed such mastery of estimation technique that he never placed a lens in the

trial frame until he was ready to test the final acuity!

With modern refractors, we can change lenses so quickly that trial and error have replaced skilled estimation. Nevertheless, situations will occur when your ability to evaluate the refractive state without lenses will be very valuable. For example, it happens commonly when screening children for ametropias, when you would like to quickly rule out large spherical errors or significant astigmatism without fussing over trial lenses or refractors.

When opacities in the ocular media obscure your view of the fundus reflex, you will find it helpful to retinoscope without the distracting reflections and reduced illumination caused by trial lenses. You will discover that estimation technique is especially useful when the reflex appears bizarre or difficult to interpret; you can move nearer to the eye for a brighter reflex and scope closer to the visual axis.

Let's look briefly at three methods for estimating the refractive error without lenses. Because you are already familiar with them, two of these techniques are easy.

When we estimate without lenses, we make four fast decisions. First, we decide whether the eye is myopic or hyperopic; then, we determine whether the eye is spheric or astigmatic; next, we locate the principal meridians; and finally, we estimate the power in these meridians.

Figure 9-1. Estimating hyper-opia in the 90° meridian by enhancing the streak reflex.

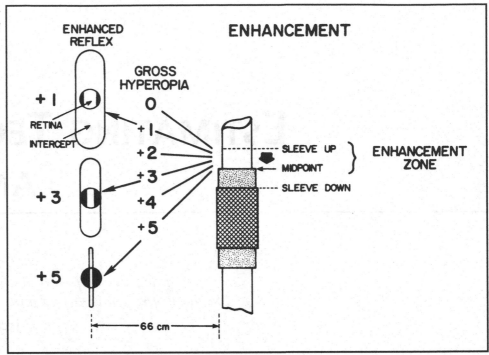

The first decision is easy: if you see WITH in both meridians (or WITH and NEUT), you can use *enhancement* for estimating the entire refractive error. Let's re-examine this familiar approach.

Exercise 47: Estimating in Low Hyperopia

We change the vergence of the beam when we lower the sleeve, and this enhances the streak reflex in WITH motion. You have used enhancement for estimating spherical hyperopia (see Figures 6-11 and 6-12) and cylinder power (see Figures 8-2 and 8-7), so now you are ready to extend the usefulness of this technique.

We will now use this familiar method (Figure 9-1) to evaluate all meridians and to locate the principal meridians and their power. We will do this by *spiraling*: rotating the streak to compare meridians while at the same time lowering the sleeve to enhance the reflex. Figure 2-7 shows how to hold the instrument for this two-handed technique. Try it.

Rx: +1.5 + 2.0 x 45.

Set your schematic eye for emmetropia at working distance (–1.5 on the corrected scale).

Place phantom –2.0s and –2.0c x 45.

At working distance, examine the reflexes. Is the eye myopic or hyperopic?

Holding the scope in both hands, *slowly* lower the sleeve while you rotate the streak. Is the eye spheric or astigmatic?

One meridian will enhance first (ie, at a higher sleeve position). This is our *spheric* meridian. Is it 45 or 135? With the streak aligned with this meridian, note the *intercept* width at this point.

Now slowly lower the sleeve further until the opposite meridian is enhanced. This is our *cylindric* meridian; note the width of the intercept now.

From the width of the intercept in the principal meridians, we can estimate the ametropia (Figure 9-2).

Your intercept at 135 should look about like +3.0 D in Figure 9-2, while the intercept at 45 is comparable to +5.0 D. Don't worry if it's imprecise since we are estimating. Do you understand why 45 looks like +5.0 D?

Our estimated gross sphere is:
+3.0s x 135 ○ +5.0s x 45.

In plus *cylinder* form this becomes:
+3.0 + 2.0c x 45, right?

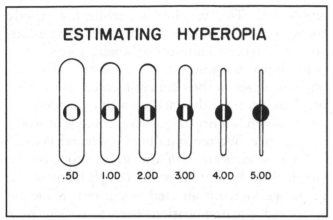

Figure 9-2. Estimating gross hyperopia. Note width of the intersection at streak enhancement in various amounts of WITH motion.

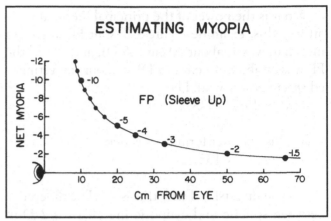

Figure 9-3. Estimating myopia by moving in to locate FPs in principal meridians. This distance from the eye to the FP indicates approximate net ametropia.

Since this is *gross*, what would the *net* be? Write it down, then compare your net with the prescription at the beginning of this exercise.

So you see that in low hyperopic ametropias such as this, we can use enhancement to make a complete spiraling estimation of the refractive error without picking up a single lens.

The spiraling technique is not useful in high hyperopia (replace the phantom sphere with a –10.0s and you will see), but that is far less common. We will deal with it later.

Going back to our first decision in estimation: what if you see AGAINST in both meridians (or AGAINST and NEUT)? This, of course, means you are sitting behind the FP; you can use the FP to estimate the ametropia, so let's look at that next.

Exercise 48: Estimating Myopia

We used the *far point location* to estimate spherical myopia (see Figure 6-10), and you will find the same method helpful in estimating myopic astigmatism without lenses (Figure 9-3).

When, for example, you see AGAINST in both meridians, you move in close to the eye with sleeve up until you have WITH in all meridians. Then recede, rotating your streak to compare meridians and locate their FPs. You will estimate the *net* error from the dioptric distance. Try it.

Rx: –5.0 + 2.0 x 135.

Remove the previous lenses. Get a ruler, or use your string or tape measure.

Readjust your eye model to corrected zero scale since this is a net technique. You may wish to recheck the zero with a working lens, then remove it.

Place a phantom +5.0s and –2.0c x 135.

Survey the reflex with the sleeve up at a working distance. It is pretty clearly AGAINST, in both meridians. Whenever you are in doubt, try the quick trick we learned earlier (p. 57): drop your sleeve to the bottom (concave mirror) to *reverse* the reflex. Now you see WITH, right? This means that it is AGAINST that you see when the sleeve is up. So, is the eye myopic or hyperopic?

With your sleeve up, move in quite close to the eye, until you see WITH in all meridians. Now recede slowly, rotating the streak to compare meridians. Keep the sleeve up. Is the eye spheric or astigmatic?

One of the meridians will begin to fill (the reflex broadens) first as you move back. Where are the principal meridians?

Is the *spheric* meridian (the FP closest to the eye, remember?) at 45 or 135? When you reach NEUT in the spheric meridian, measure the distance from your forehead to the protractor on the model eye with a ruler. Is it about 20 cm (8 inches)? Be careful to maintain optical alignment while measuring the FP. If you use a string on the scope handle, add 2 to 3 cm for the extra distance to the peephole.

Now recede further and find the FP in the *cylindric* meridian. Is it located at about 33 cm (13 inches)?

What is the power of the principal meridians? To answer this, examine Figure 9-3. Our FP in the 45 meridian was at about 20 cm (–5 D), and at 135 the FP was at about 33 cm (–3 D). So, our net estimated *sphere* power would be:

–5.0s x 45 $\backsim$ –3.0s x 135.

In plus cylinder form, this is net:

–5.0 + 2.0c x 135.

Do you understand why this is so? The difference between spheric and cylindric meridians is 2 D in the "plus direction," hence +2.0c.

What would be the *gross* neutralizing lens at 66 cm? Calculate this before proceeding.

Place a –3.5s and a +2.0c x 135 before the schematic eye. Do you see NEUT at working distance?

The gross (excluding phantoms) is:

–3.5 +2.0c x 135.

So (deducting 1.5 D), the *net* would be:

–5.0 +2.0 x 135

This is where we came in. Notice the different relationship of gross to net in myopia.

Try this method once again on your own. Have your helper create an unknown compound myopic astigmatism using any moderate (+3 to +5 D) sphere phantom with a phantom cylinder (–1 to –3 D) on any axis. Use your left eye to estimate the net error. See how close you can come to the phantom net. Now write your correction as the gross.

So much for the familiar methods of estimating without lenses. Now let's try something a little complex.

Estimating by Direct Retinoscopy

Copeland described an estimating method he referred to as "ophthalmoscopic retinoscopy." In this technique, you hold the retinoscope close to the patient's eye (as with an ophthalmoscope) while looking for the image of the bulb *filament* focused on the retina (retinoscopic focus). I prefer to call this method *direct retinoscopy*, for we are seeking an image inside the eye, as opposed to *indirect* (FP) methods where we view an image in the retinoscope. This terminology, while not strictly correct optically, provides instructive comparisons vis-à-vis direct and indirect ophthalmoscopy.

In direct retinoscopy, we seek the sharpest, brightest image of the filament focused on the retina. Do not confuse this method with enhancing the reflex, which is a neutralization technique at working distance. We use spiraling (combined vertical and rotary movement of the sleeve) to compare meridians as before. As in direct ophthalmoscopy, the image we see is affected by our own refractive error and accommodation (our focus on near objects). It is natural to accommodate excessively when trying to find the clearest image, especially when working up close to the eye. Beware: this can affect your endpoint. Try to relax your focus, as if you were gazing at the horizon.

Fragments of direct retinoscopy appear in Copeland's descriptions of estimating techniques. Weinstock and Wirtschafter[1] later put the pieces together, replacing the individual maneuvers with a single, unified movement diagram, which you can hang on the wall beside your refracting chair (Figure 9-4). The technique is especially helpful when the reflex is aberrated or dull and in aphakia and other high ametropias.

You begin with the sleeve up, 5 cm (2 inches) from the eye. Without moving backward, spiral the sleeve slowly downward, rotating the streak to compare meridians as you search for the filament focus on the retina. If you find no focus when the sleeve has reached bottom (maximum concave mirror), slowly recede from the eye while continuing to rotate the streak. When you first find the filament focus, measure the distance to the eye; determine the approximate *net* power in that meridian from the scale (see Figure 9-4).

When you first see the filament focus, that meridian is the *spheric*. If the focus is the same in the opposite meridian, determine the power from the scale, and you are done. If the filament is not focused in the opposite (*cylindric*) meridian, you continue on with the movement until you find the focus, then locate the power on the scale. As luck (and optics) would have it, this second meridian is the axis of the plus cylinder. If you do not find the second focus, start all over again; you may have missed one the first time.

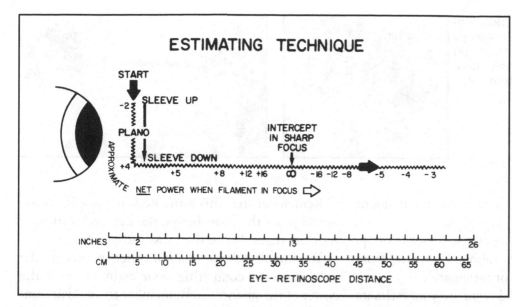

Figure 9-4. Movement pattern for estimating with direct retinoscopy, using approximate calibrations for Copeland-type instruments. The jagged line indicates rotation of the streak (Adapted from Weinstock SM, Wirtschafter JD. *A Decision-Oriented Manual of Retinoscopy.* Springfield, Ill: Charles C. Thomas; 1976).

In the diagram, you see that the intercept is in sharp focus (on the protractor of schematic eye or refractor) when you are 30 to 35 cm (about 13 inches) from the eye. This serves nicely to separate myopic from hyperopic ametropias. In fact, only about 6 cm separates +18 from –18 D, so if the filament is in focus about a foot from the eye, it is important to note whether this is before the intercept (+18), or after (–18). The movement pattern is similar, but the scale calibration is somewhat different in retinoscopes that converge the beam with the sleeve up. If you have one of these non-Copeland instruments, you should examine the appropriate diagram.[1]

So much for how it works. Let's put it to the test with a few examples that you should enjoy.

Exercise 49: Emmetropia

Your model eye should be at zero on the corrected scale.

Move in to 5 cm from the eye with your sleeve up. The filament on the "retina" is out of focus, correct?

Slowly spiral the sleeve downward. Does the filament come into sharp focus with the sleeve about halfway down? Compare this with the plano location in the diagram. It works!

Try this method on your partner or helper, with his or her correcting lenses (if any) in place. Is the image sharp with the sleeve about halfway down (assuming emmetropia)?

Exercise 50: High Hyperopia (Aphakia)

Now add a –10.0s phantom to the schematic eye.

Start over, at 5 cm with the sleeve up. You will see that the filament is completely out of focus.

Spiral the sleeve downward to the bottom. Is the image still fuzzy?

Now slowly move away from the eye until the filament is in sharp focus. Is this at about 20 to 25 cm (9 inches)? You will notice that the endpoint (the sharpest, brightest image) is a little vague; don't fret, we are estimating. At least you know the approximate power.

Is the focus the same in all meridians? Measure your endpoint distance and compare with the power scale in Figure 9-4. Are you close?

Exercise 51: High Myopia

Replace the phantom with a +10.0s.

Repeat your search for the filament focus; start close with the sleeve up. Use your left eye.

Spiral downward until the sleeve reaches bottom. Now begin moving back while rotating the streak. It is important to remain close while spiraling down, receding only *after* the sleeve reaches bottom. When you get to 30 to 35 cm (about 13 inches) from the eye, you will see that the intercept is now focused on the protractor or pupil, while the filament on the retina is still blurred. Recall that the intercept focus separates high hyperopia from

Figure 9-5. Preliminary estimation with direct (ophthalmoscopic) retinoscopy using refractor. (A) Starting at 5 cm. (B) Receding while rotating streak. Note hand positions for Optec instrument.

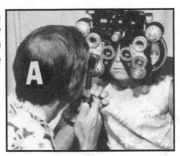
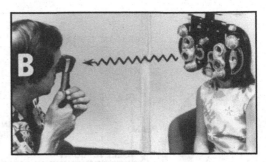

high myopia. Since you have not seen the filament focus yet, you do not have hyperopia.

Continue to move back until the image is sharp. This should be 40 to 45 cm (about 17 inches) from the eye. Is the eye spheric or astigmatic?

Measure the distance and compare your estimate with the scale.

Exercise 52: Hyperopic Astigmatism

We will try one example of astigmatism to show how this method works when there are two principal meridians.

Replace the phantom with a –4.0s and a –2.0c x 180.

Follow the movements in the diagram as before; start very close with the sleeve up.

Remember to spiral slowly, lowering the sleeve while rotating the streak. Relax your accommodation. Is this a spherical ametropia?

What is the height of the sleeve when the filament image first comes into sharp focus? Which meridian focuses first?

While you are at 5 cm, the image should first appear in the 90 meridian, when the sleeve is at the bottom. Does yours? Check Figure 9-4. What is the approximate power at this point?

Now recede with the sleeve down and find the focus in the opposite meridian. Is this at 15 to 18 cm (about 6 or 7 inches)?

From the scale, you would guess the power at this point to be about +6 D or more. So our estimate would be:

+4.0s x 90 ∽ +6.0s x 180.

In plus cylinder form this becomes:
+4.0 + 2.0c x 180.

Remember that this estimate is *net* power, so you would place the gross before the eye and start neutralizing there. Write the gross (answer below*).

You might wish to try a few other spherocylinder combinations, comparing your estimate with the power of the phantoms. Remember to avoid accommodating, or you will alter the filament image and thus your endpoint.

Retinoscope your assistant again, this time without his or her correcting lenses. If he or she is emmetropic, find someone who is not. Is the eye myopic or hyperopic? Spheric or astigmatic? What are the principal meridians? What is their approximate power? Figure 9-5 illustrates the technique.

The linear measurements are difficult, and the estimates are occasionally misleading (especially in low myopia). Direct retinoscopy is a valuable technique for getting your bearings when you are really lost in hazy media or aberrations of the reflex. It is worth reemphasizing that the intercept separates high hyperopia from high myopia, which, in itself, makes this technique a useful tool.

Remember that the scale of the movement pattern represents a composite of how several Copeland-type retinoscopes focus. Every instrument is a little different; if the technique appeals to you, make your own calibration scale using phantom lenses.

Once mastered, some students find this approach to be really useful; they employ it for a preliminary survey of the reflex in every patient. Others find direct retinoscopy only occasionally helpful since most ametropias (which cluster between +2 and –3 D) can be easily recognized and neutralized without the need for preliminary estimations.

If you do not use this direct technique, you will lose it. Practice it periodically on cooperative patients when time permits. Keep a copy of the pat-

*+5.50 + 2.0c x 180.

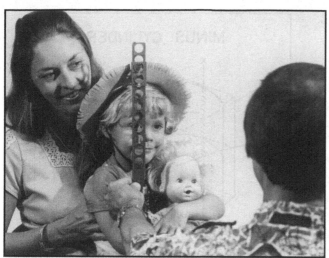

Figure 9-6. Estimating with a lens rack. You watch the reflex while rapidly passing a wide range of spheres before the eye from a non-threatening distance. Here we use the neutralizing-with-spheres method (see Figure 7-8).

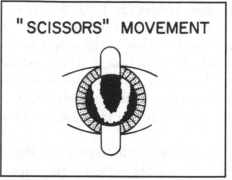

Figure 9-7. Scissors motion. As the streak passes across the pupil, we see two reflex bands, which appear to open and close like blades of a scissors.

tern (see Figure 9-4) with your scope; the day will come when you will need it.

With estimating techniques, you can have fun with your retinoscope at home without lenses. Practice on your family and on anyone who comes to call; children and dogs are especially good subjects.

With infants and young children, where estimation is most needed, direct retinoscopy is not as helpful as you might expect because they usually will not cooperate for the working distances and measurements required. Since they are usually hyperopic, you usually can estimate ametropias in small children better by enhancing (see Figures 6-11 and 6-12) or with a retinoscopy lens rack (Figure 9-6); both techniques allow you to keep your distance and are not much affected by squirming.

Remember that estimating techniques are, after all, merely shortcuts to determine the approximate refractive error. You must confirm your findings by neutralizing whenever possible.

RELIABILITY AND ACCURACY

Retinoscopy is an extremely precise and accurate optical measuring technique under ideal circumstances, like you might find in a properly calibrated schematic eye. Unfortunately, these ideal circum-

stances seldom exist in refracting lanes, so we accept a certain amount of predictable error and, whenever possible, we ask the patient to verify our measurements. Discrepancies between our objective findings and the patient's subjective refinement arise from several sources: from the patient's eye, from our technique, and from our interpretations of the endpoints. While we can control some of these sources of error to a certain extent, others (being in the nature of optics) are uncontrollable.

In the normal eye itself, *spherical aberration* (see Figure 4-17) and *irregular astigmatism* (both pronounced when the pupil is dilated) produce varying degrees of *optical turbulence*. Much of this turbulence goes unnoticed (especially with a small pupil), but occasionally irregular reflexes, swirls, and *scissors motion* will be truly troublesome (Figure 9-7).

When you confront these bizarre reflexes, change from the *indirect* (neutralizing) technique to the *direct* (estimating) method. Turbulence is most confusing near NEUT, so by moving in close on axis without distracting lenses, you may save the day. Occasionally (especially in keratoconus or corneal scarring) objective methods simply will not work and you will have to switch to trial-and-error subjective testing.

Chromatic (color) *aberration* and *coma* (spherical aberration of oblique rays) create discrepancies between the objective and subjective sphere power that are beyond your control. On the other hand, you can usually control *accommodation* (contraction of the ciliary muscle, which increases the power of the patient's lens) with fogging methods and nonaccommodative targets (p. 108). When you cannot control accommodation (as in children, young hyperopes and certain uptight persons), you will occasionally find *cycloplegic* drops (which briefly paralyze the ciliary muscle) necessary to prevent huge sphere errors. Unfortunately these drugs also dilate the pupil, thus reintroducing other sources of error.

Your technique itself, especially *alignment* and *distance*, predictably affects the accuracy of retinoscopy. Incorrect optical alignment produces *radial astigmatism*, which distorts the cylinder power and to a lesser extent the sphere. It is not possible to retinoscope right on the visual axis unless the patient is looking directly at your scope; without cycloplegia, this induces accommodation errors and miosis (reduced pupil size). With a dilated pupil, however, spherical aberration creeps in. So try to stay as close to the axis as possible, and avoid cycloplegics. If the pupil is dilated, watch the reflex in the very center. Errors in working distance or its allowance (in correcting gross to net) can cause you to misjudge the power of the sphere, as you well know.

Errors in your subjective *interpretation* of the endpoints are especially difficult to control, and sometimes even to recognize. Judging neutrality or the quality of meridians takes a lot of experience. By analyzing the patient's acceptance or rejection of your findings, you will continually improve your accuracy. At first, some patients won't see "the big E" with your retinoscopy; don't be discouraged, it has happened to us all.

As you gain experience, ask yourself *why* your refraction was rejected. After a year of self-evaluation you may be able to say: "I tend to overplus the sphere" or "I'm poor at refining the axis." This knowledge will improve your reliability and accuracy and teach you when to give more (or less) weight to the patient's preference when it differs from your measurements. Occasionally, we all come up with retinoscopy findings that are very misleading, and the reasons for this error seem to escape analysis. Well, nothing is perfect.

By comparing the objective and subjective refraction, we can analyze retinoscopy in terms of *precision* (repeatability), *accuracy* (freedom from error), and *bias* (the tendency to err in a particular direction).[2]

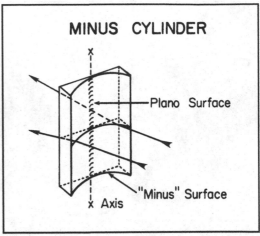

Figure 9-8. A minus cylinder (planoconcave) placed with axis vertical. The concave (power) surface diverges arriving rays. The plano surface (axis meridian) has no power. Compare with Figure 3-11.

Studies of experienced retinoscopists found that they measured cylinder power more precisely and accurately than sphere power, and right eyes (!) more precisely than left eyes. Analysis for bias shows retinoscopy tends to overestimate hyperopia and the power of the cylinder, while underestimating myopia. Statistical evaluation of experienced practitioners also demonstrates an interesting degree of variability. Some retinoscopists are very precise but inaccurate, while others are accurate but imprecise.[3,4]

Overall, it is safe to say that *retinoscopy* is most accurate for cylinder axis, moderately accurate for cylinder power, and least accurate for sphere. Conversely, *subjective* refinement is best for sphere, good for cylinder power, and worst for cylinder axis. In other words, the most accurate measurements are the objective cylinder and the subjective sphere. This is why careful retinoscopy, refined by the patient, makes the most reliable prescription.

MINUS CYLINDER RETINOSCOPY

Just as peanut butter goes with jelly, plus cylinders complement retinoscopy. But we can modify our technique so that we can use *minus cylinders* when necessary (Figure 9-8).

Minus cylinders act the opposite of plus cylinders (ie, they *diverge* light rays arriving along the power meridian). Since the vergence of the cylinder is

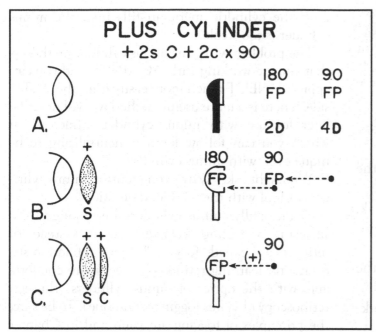

Figure 9-9. Plus cylinder method. (A) The 180 meridian (FP closest to the eye) is the spheric; the 90 meridian (furthest FP) is the cylindric. (B) The sphere (+2s) moves both meridians until the closest FP (180) is NEUT. (C) The plus cylinder (+2c) moves only the furthest FP (90) until it is NEUT.

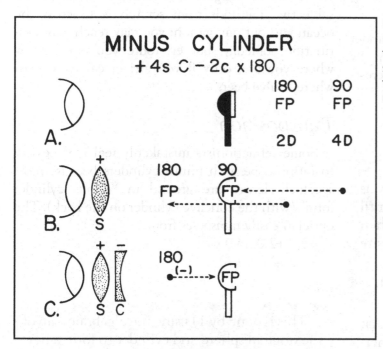

Figure 9-10. Minus cylinder method. (A) The 90 meridian (FP furthest from the eye) is the spheric; the 180 meridian (closest FP) is the cylinder. (B) The sphere (+4s) moves both meridians until the furthest FP (90) is NEUT. (C) The minus cylinder (−2c) moves only the closest FP (180) until it is NEUT.

reversed, we *must treat the emerging FPs in reverse order* when we neutralize with minus cylinders. We first neutralize the FP *furthest* from the eye with our sphere, the FP *closest* to the eye with our minus cylinder. These spheric and cylindric meridians are just the opposite of those we described in Table 7-1. Figures 9-9 and 9-10 illustrate the differences between the two methods. The ametropia (SHA) is the same in both cases, but the meridians are han-

dled quite differently. Study and compare the diagrams, to be sure you understand this. Take note how the same correcting prescription appears when written in plus and minus cylinder form.

How would you go about neutralizing if you only had minus cylinders? The *minus cylinder method* (with schematic eye or trial frame) consists of these steps:

Minus Cylinder Method:

1. Evaluate reflexes with sleeve up at working distance.

2. Convert all meridians to AGAINST using spheres.

3. Reduce sphere, comparing meridians until one meridian is NEUT.

4. Apply minus cylinder to neutralize the opposite meridian.

5. Move in and out a little, rotating streak, to compare meridians. Refine if necessary.

6. Check working distance. Result is the gross refraction.

7. Reduce sphere (only) by dioptric working distance to achieve net.

Compare these steps with the plus cylinder method on page 68. We will not dwell on this by doing any exercises, but for those who are interested, this is how to handle the reflexes.

Simplified Minus Cylinder Method:

1. Both reflexes are WITH (CHA).
   Add plus spheres until both meridians are AGAINST, then reduce plus until first (spheric) meridian is NEUT. Then add minus cylinder to the opposite meridian.

2. One reflex is WITH (SHA, MIX-A).
   Proceed exactly as in (1) above.

3. Neither reflex is WITH (SMA, CMA).
   Add minus spheres until the first (spheric) meridian is NEUT, then add minus cylinder to the opposite meridian.

You may wish to compare this procedure with that for plus cylinders (page 71). When refining the cylinder axis (straddling), we move a minus cylinder *away* from the guide line. We refine the cylinder power by *minus cylinder rules*: 1) if the spheric meridian fills first, the minus cylinder is too strong;

2) if the cylindric meridian fills first, the minus cylinder is too weak.

The problem with this minus cylinder method is that you are working with AGAINST, and you can approach NEUT much more easily from the WITH side. There is a more useful method we will describe later for use with minus cylinder refractors, in which you can follow familiar neutralizing technique even with minus cylinders.

You might ask, "Why even mention minus cylinders or fool with them?" Good question.

Traditionally, minus cylinders are required for a *subjective refracting technique* (used instead of retinoscopy) called "fogging."[5] Many refractionists, even after learning retinoscopy, feel more comfortable with the optics of minus cylinders (through retinoscopy obviates fogging technique). To be sure, the principles of fogging are valid and in Chapter 13 we will use fogging *after* retinoscopy. But to use subjective methods from scratch is to cross the ocean without navigation: you may reach your destination someday, but en route you don't know where you are; only if you arrive, can you guess where you've been.

Transposition

Some refractionists mistakenly feel it necessary to retinoscope with minus cylinders because most spectacle lenses are ground in "minus cylinder form" (with the concave cylinder on the back). The optician easily *transposes* from:

+2.0 +2.0 x 90 to
+4.0 –2.0 x 180

This is done by 1) using the algebraic sum of the original sphere and cylinder to form a new sphere; then 2) reversing the sign of the cylinder (keeping its power the same); while, 3) rotating the axis 90°. It's only numbers. Thus: –2.0 + 2.0 x 90 becomes plano –2.0 x 180.

You will need to know transposition, so review the prescription in Figures 9-9 and 9-10 to be sure you understand the mechanism.

You need familiarity with minus cylinders only to be able to use a minus cylinder refractor if you are given no alternative. The simplest minus cylinder method, which prevents the confusion inherent in reversing all your techniques, is called the "double-click" method.[3] It is described on page 120.

Despite my bias in favor of plus cylinder techniques as taught by Copeland, minus cylinder refractors work best with minus cylinder techniques (see Chapter 10 for these techniques).

In the final chapter, we will discuss the best methods for putting into practice what you have learned.

REFERENCES

1. Weinstock SM, Wirtschafter JD. *A Decision-Oriented Manual of Retinoscopy.* Springfield, Ill: Charles C. Thomas; 1976:6,99.

2. Hyams L, Safir, A. Statistical concepts in refraction. *Int Ophthalmol Clin.* 1971;11:103-114.

3. Safir A, Hyams L, Philpot J, et al. Studies in refraction: I. The precision of retinoscopy. *Arch Ophthalmol.* 1970;84:49-61.

4. Hyams L, Safir A, Philpot J. Studies in refraction: II. Bias and accuracy of retinoscopy. *Arch Ophthalmol.* 1971;85:22-41.

5. Sloane AE, ed. *Manual of Refraction.* 2nd ed. Boston, Mass: Little, Brown and Co; 1970:117.

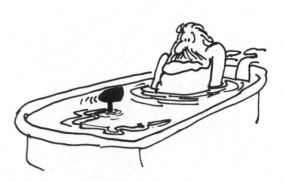

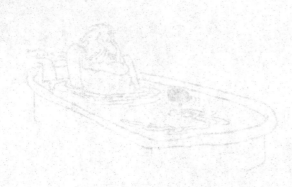

MINUS CYLINDER RETINOSCOPY

David J. Norath, COT

"Why would you want to retinoscope with minus cylinders?!"

Jack Copeland

Neutralizing in minus cylinder is relatively no different than neutralizing in plus cylinder. It is a matter of which principal meridian you choose to neutralize first. With astigmatism, there are always two principal meridians: the spherical meridian and the cylinder meridian. I always recommend neutralizing the sphere first and the cylinder second.

The approach for neutralizing in minus cylinder is this: start your retinoscopy by determining the two principal meridians and analyze which meridian has the greatest plus or least minus. This meridian will be the spherical meridian. Once this is neutralized, proceed to neutralize the second meridian (which should be against motion). At the second meridian, since one sees AGAINST motion, add minus cylinder at the same axis you are scoping until neutralization is found. If you see WITH motion in the second meridian, simply start over at that meridian by neutralizing the sphere, and then go 90° away to neutralize the cylinder. The two principal meridians are always 90° away from each other. Here are all the possibilities you will see initially when doing retinoscopy on a person with astigmatism:

First, think of the possibilities as though they are on a number line. Since we are working in minus cylinder, work from right to left (Figure 10-1).

INITIAL ANALYSIS OF THE TWO PRINCIPAL MERIDIANS

- First meridian (+) and the second meridian (+) is compound hyperopic astigmatism.
- First meridian (+) and the second meridian 0 is simple hyperopic astigmatism.
- First meridian 0 and the second meridian (–) is simple myopic astigmatism.
- First meridian (–) and the second meridian (–) is compound myopic astigmatism.
- First meridian (+) and the second meridian (–) is mixed astigmatism.

Let's quickly review the basic steps of retinoscopy before we start our approach to neutralizing using minus cylinder. Position yourself 26 inches from the patient. Hold the sleeve of the retinoscope in the up position if using the Optec 360 Streak Retinoscope or sleeve down if using a Welch Allyn. This will produce plano mirror effect. If you're not sure how the sleeve is placed (up or down), simply hold your hand in front of the retinoscope about 5 or 6 inches. The beam of light projected should be fat and wide, as opposed to narrow and skinny. Place the "R" lens in your phoropter or use a +1.50 sph in a trial frame. The "R" lens is equal to +1.50

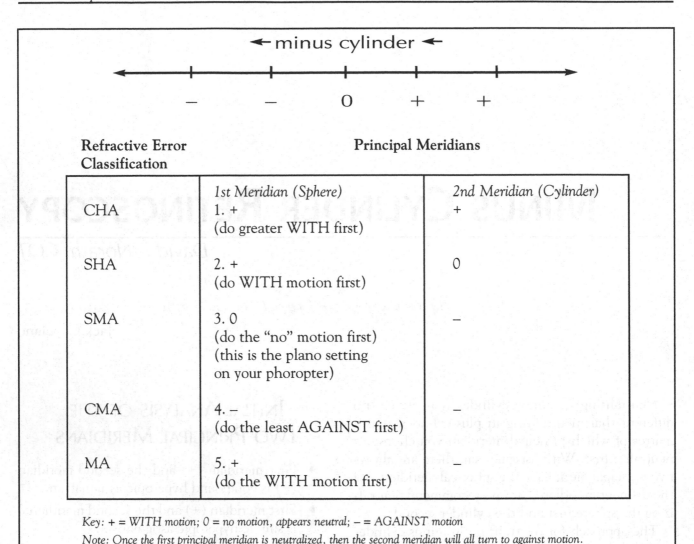

Figure 10-1. Schematic approach to neutralizing reflexes using minus cylinders.

sph unless the doctor special ordered a stronger lens for the phoropter. Some technicians prefer not to use a "R" lens and simply subtract a +1.50 sph from the end results of the sphere.

Determine the principal meridians: WITH motion add plus or move in a plus direction of travel, or AGAINST motion add minus or move in a minus direction of travel. Neutralize the sphere first by using spherical lenses on your phoropter or in your trial lens set. Make sure the first meridian is neutralized before proceeding to neutralize the second meridian (90° away from the first meridian). The second meridian is then neutralized with cylinder setting the axis at the same meridian that you are scoping.

There are three tests to verify neutralization:

1. **Move in and move out.** If you feel you have the spherical meridian neutralized, move in closer with your retinoscope to about 13 inches and see WITH motion, then move out beyond your 26 inches to about 39 inches and see AGAINST motion.

2. **Play "the price is right."** Example: If the patient actually looks neutralized with a +1.00 sph try a +2.00 sph and see AGAINST motion, and then try a plano lens and see WITH motion. In other words, go above and below the neutral lens to set limits. This will be especially helpful when doing your refractometry. If the patient goes beyond these limits, then you know the patient's responses are not reliable.

3. **Reverse the sleeve of the retinoscope.** In using the Optec 360 streak retinoscope, if it is neutralized with sleeve up, it will be neutralized with sleeve down. If you see any kind of movement by reversing the sleeve re-analyze with the sleeve in the up position. By dropping the sleeve of the retinoscope down one creates concave mirror effect and what was WITH motion with the sleeve up is now AGAINST motion with the sleeve down. In other words, every movement is reversed.

If it's neutralized with sleeve up it will be neutralized with sleeve down. To obtain concave mirror effect with the Welch Allyn raise the sleeve up, and for the Welch Allyn, if it's neutralized with sleeve down, it will be neutralized with sleeve up. There is actually a fourth way to verify neutralization and I call it *drop back and punt.* If you see neutralization, reverse the sleeve of your retinoscope and move out to about 39 inches and see WITH motion. Make sure the spherical meridian is neutralized using the three tests to verify neutralization. Otherwise, if the spherical meridian isn't neutralized properly, this will throw the amount of cylinder correction off by the amount of power not corrected in the spherical meridian.

After the spherical meridian is neutralized, proceed to the second meridian, which will always be 90° away from the first meridian by rotating the sleeve of your retinoscope. The second meridian is the cylinder meridian. Add cylinder at the same axis that you are scoping until neutralization is found, and use the three tests to verify neutralization, the same way that you did the spherical meridian.

PRACTICE EXAMPLES USING A SCHEMATIC EYE AND TRIAL LENSES: NEUTRALIZING IN MINUS CYLINDER

The schematic eye that I use in the examples is an English-made schematic eye that can be purchased from Western Ophthalmics (catalog number WO-109, see p. 46). Set the schematic eye to the "zero" setting by pulling the back portion outward. Scope the schematic eye at 26 inches, and see if it is neutralized with no lenses placed in front. This schematic eye is made to work without using a

working distance lens of +1.50 sph. If the schematic eye is not neutralized at the "zero" setting, adjust it accordingly. If you are still seeing WITH motion, pull the back of the schematic eye outward slightly until neutralized. If you are seeing AGAINST motion, push the back of the schematic eye inward, until neutralized.

Make sure you use the *three tests to verify neutralization*:

1. Move in and see WITH motion and move out and see AGAINST motion.

2. Play the price is right by placing a +.50 sph in front of the schematic eye and see AGAINST motion. Then remove that lens and place a .50 sph in front of the schematic eye to see WITH motion, and then remove that lens.

3. Reverse the sleeve of the retinoscope. IF it's neutralized with sleeve up, it will be neutralized with sleeve down (using the Optec 360 Streak retinoscope). Using the Welch Allyn retinoscope, if it's neutralized with sleeve down, it will be neutralized with sleeve up.

Remember, reversing the sleeve of the retinoscope creates a concave mirror effect that will cause one to see the exact opposite of what one sees when the sleeve is in plano mirror effect. *The opposite of neutralization is neutralization.* Usually this type of schematic eye can be off by .25 to .50 D. Note your setting, in case you accidentally bump the back of your schematic eye, while practicing the following examples.

Example 1: Compound Hyperopic Astigmatism

Place a –1.50 sph and a –1.50 cylinder x 90° in the slots closest to your neutralized schematic eye. These phantom lenses are used to create the refractive error. Now, forget about those lenses that were placed in the schematic eye and begin your retinoscopy without using a +1.50 sph working lens. Remember the schematic eye was calibrated to work without the "R" lens or the +1.50 sph working lens.

When beginning your retinoscopy, establish your two principal meridians. This will be the 180° and the 90° meridians. The two principal meridians are determined by how the streak of your retinoscope aligns itself by using the break phenomenon, the brightness phenomenon, and the skew phenomenon. Notice that in both meridians one will see WITH motion, but there will be more WITH motion at the 90° than at 180° meridian. Remember, when working in minus cylinder we want to neutralize the greatest WITH motion first, which will be the 90° meridian. Begin neutralizing the 90° meridian with spherical lenses trying +1.00 D spherical steps. Try a +1.00 sph and still see WITH motion. Then try a +2.00 sph and still see WITH. Finally, try a +3.00 sph and this looks neutralized. Try a +3.50 sph and see AGAINST motion. Therefore, you will need to go back to the +3.00 sph. This is one way to make sure the +3.00 sph is the correct lens for neutralization ("playing the price is right"). Move in and see WITH motion, and then move out beyond your 26-inch working distance and see AGAINST motion. Reverse the sleeve of the retinoscope, and see neutralization in both plano mirror effect and concave mirror effect.

Now that we have the sphere neutralized and checked ways to verify neutralization, proceed to rotate the sleeve of the retinoscope to the 180° meridian, leaving the spherical lens in your schematic eye. At the 180° meridian, one will now see AGAINST motion. If you have a hard time trying to see the AGAINST motion, reverse the sleeve of the retinoscope and see WITH motion, this will confirm the AGAINST motion that one sees in the plano mirror effect. At the same axis that you are scoping, add minus cylinder in 1.00 D steps, the same way that you neutralized the sphere. Try a −1.00 cylinder at 180°: this will then look a little AGAINST. Try a −2.00 cylinder at 180° and see WITH motion ("playing the price is right"). Therefore, the selected lens should be between a −1.00 and a −2.00, which is a −1.50 cylinder x 180°. Place the −1.50 cylinder x 180° in your schematic eye and proceed to do the other two ways to verify neutralization: move in to about 13 inches and see WITH motion and move out beyond your 26 inch working distance to about 39 inches and see AGAINST motion, go back to your working distance of 26 inches and reverse the sleeve of the retinoscope and see neutralization in both plano mirror effect and concave mirror effect. The final prescription will read +3.00 sph −1.50 cyl x 180°.

Example 2: Simple Hyperopic Astigmatism (SHA)

Place a −1.50 cylinder x 90° in the slot closest to your neutralized schematic eye. This phantom lens is used to create the refractive error. Now, forget about this lens that was placed in the schematic eye and begin your retinoscopy without using a +1.50 sph working lens. Remember the schematic eye was calibrated to work without the "R" lens or the +1.50 sph working lens.

When beginning your retinoscopy, establish your two principal meridians. This will be the 180° and 90° meridians. The two principal meridians are determined by how the streak of your retinoscope aligns itself by using the break phenomenon, the brightness phenomenon, and the skew phenomenon. Notice in one meridian (at axis 90°), one will see WITH motion and in the 180° meridian one will see "no" motion or NEUT. Therefore, in this example we want to neutralize the 90° meridian first. This will neutralize using a +1.50 sph lens. Do the three tests to verify neutralization at 90° meridian first. This will neutralize using a +1.50 sph lens. Do the three tests to verify neutralization at 90°, then proceed to the 180° meridian to neutralize the cylinder. Since you see AGAINST motion at the 180° meridian, add minus cylinder at the same axis that you are scoping until the meridian looks neutral. Then proceed to verify neutralization by doing the three tests to verify neutralization. The final prescription will read +1.50 sph −1.50 cyl x 180°.

Example 3: Simple Myopic Astigmatism

Place a +1.50 cylinder x 90° in the slot closest to your neutralized schematic eye. This phantom lens is once again used to create the refractive error. Now, forget about this lens that was placed in the schematic eye, and begin your retinoscopy.

Establish your two principal meridians. This will be 90° and 180°. At 90° you will see AGAINST motion and at 180° it will look neutral. Do the 180° meridian first, and this will neutralize with a plano lens. Do the 3 tests to verify neutralization at 180° before proceeding to do the cylinder. Next, neutralize the 90° meridian by placing minus cylinder at the same axis that you are scoping. This will neutralize with a –1.50 cylinder x 90°. Do the 3 tests to verify neutralization. The final prescription will read: Plano –1.50 cyl x 90°.

Example 4: Compound Myopic Astigmatism (CMA)

Place a +1.50 sph and a +1.50 cylinder x 90° in the slots of your schematic eye. These phantom lenses are used to create the refractive error. Now, forget about these lenses, and begin your retinoscopy.

Establish your two principal meridians, which will be 90° and 180°. You will see AGAINST motion in both meridians. Do the least amount of AGAINST first. This will be 180°. The 180° meridian will neutralize with a –1.50 sph. Do the three tests to verify neutralization at 180° before proceeding to do the 90° meridian.

Now that the 180° meridian is neutralized with a –1.50 sph, leave that lens in there and proceed to neutralize the cylinder at 90°. Since you see AGAINST motion, add minus cylinder at the same axis you are scoping until it appears neutralized. If you add too much minus cylinder you will start to see WITH motion. Do the three tests to verify neutralization. The final prescription will read: –1.50 sph –1.50 cyl x 90°.

Example 5: Mixed Astigmatism (MIX-A)

Place a –1.50 sph and a + 2.50 cylinder x 90° in the slots of your schematic eye. These phantom lenses are used to create the refractive error. Now, disregard these lenses, and begin your retinoscopy.

Establish your two principal meridians, which will be 90° and 180°. You will see AGAINST motion at 90° and WITH motion at 180°. Neutralize the WITH motion first with a spherical lens at 180°. This will neutralize with a +1.50 sph. Do the three tests to verify neutralization, then proceed to the 90° meridian to neutralize the cylinder. Since you see AGAINST motion add minus cylinder at the same axis that you are scoping (90°). This meridian will neutralize with a –2.50 cylinder x 90°. Repeat the three tests to again verify neutralization.

The final prescription will read: +150 sph –2.50 cyl x 90°.

In the preceding examples, we used the 90° and the 180° meridians for simplicity. However, when you actually do a real eye the two principal meridians can be anywhere. Just remember that the two principal meridians are always 90° apart from each other. So, if the one principal meridian is 10°, the other principal meridian will be 100°. Also, keep in mind that our eyes are usually symmetrical. For example, if one eye has astigmatism at 90°, it will usually be 90° in the other eye; and if at 180°, it will usually be 180° in the other eye. If the cylinder lies nasally on one eye, it will usually be nasally on the other eye; and if out temporally on one eye, it will usually be temporally on the other eye. Is it possible to have astigmatism at 90° in one eye and 180° in the other? Yes, but double-check to make sure. This is especially true in cases in which the patient had cataract surgery with lens implantation

When doing real eyes, place the "R" lenses in front of both eyes to avoid the patient looking at the occluder and stimulating accommodation. This is especially important if the patient isn't cyclopleged. Have the patient look at the red-green filter with no letters. This will limit the usual white reflections that one sees when doing retinoscopy. Therefore, I suggest you don't use the big "E" or white fixation dot, and never have the patient look at the light of your retinoscope. This will create a glare and you will have a hard time seeing the reflex.

Aligning your streak to the patient's eye is very important. Therefore, scope right eye to patient's right eye, and left eye to patient's left eye. What happens if you have only one good eye and the other eye is amblyopic or blind? Then, simply use your same good eye to scope each patient's eye. If you are not aligned properly, this could induce some astigmatism that isn't really there. You can maintain alignment if you note small white dots that are projected from your retinoscope, called the Purkinje reflexes. If you see two small white dot reflections, move horizontally and/or vertically until the two dots are superimposed centrally. Once this is achieved, you are then properly aligned with the patient's eye reflex (see Figure 5-7).

You can practice retinoscopy on those patients seeing 20/20 with their present glasses. Simply check the patient's visual acuity to confirm 20/20, then check the patient's glasses. Your retinoscopy results should be similar to the patient's glasses (if not exactly the same). Just like any skill that one learns, with practice and time one will become very proficient in retinoscopy.

CONCAVE MIRROR RETINOSCOPY

David J. Norath, COT

"You can see a lot just by looking!"
"Yogi" Berra

Earlier (pp. 57-58), we described a concave mirror test to assist in evaluating the frequently puzzling AGAINST reflex. Here is an amplification of those techniques for advanced students.

For high myopic patients it is often difficult to see the AGAINST motion. You sweep the streak of the retinoscope all the way on and off the pupil of the patient's eye, but the AGAINST motion that you see doesn't occur until the streak is halfway across the patient's pupil. To make it easier to see the AGAINST motion, try reversing the sleeve of the retinoscope. In other words, reverse the sleeve to the concave mirror position. With Copeland-types, this would mean sleeve down. When you see the WITH reflex in the concave mirror position, you know that the motion you were seeing in the plano mirror position was the exact opposite, or AGAINST motion. You may then add minus lenses until the WITH motion is neutralized. Again, placing the sleeve in the concave mirror position will give the exact opposite of what one sees in the plano mirror position. So if you saw WITH motion in the plano mirror position, the reflex will be AGAINST in the concave mirror position. Also, if you see neutralization in the plano mirror effect, then it will be neutral in the concave mirror effect. (see Figures 2-4 and 2-5 for the optics of sleeve positioning).

EXAMPLE 1:
SEEING WITH IN THE CONCAVE MIRROR POSITION, SIMPLE MYOPIA

Set the schematic eye, such as the Western Ophthalmics (WO-109), in a –3.00 diopter position by pulling the schematic eye outward to create the "long" eye of myopia. Position yourself at the normal working distance (26 inches). First, look at the reflex in the plano mirror position (sleeve up using the Optec 360 and sleeve down using the Welch Allyn). Note that the AGAINST motion is puzzling. Now, reverse the sleeve of the retinoscope (concave mirror effect) and see WITH motion. Add minus spherical power (the opposite of what you'd do to neutralize WITH motion in the plane mirror position), until the reflex is neutralized. Note that if you chose to neutralize the 90° meridian first, you would then check the 180° meridian second, to see if astigmatism is present. In this example all meridians will be neutralized with a –3.00 sphere, so the refractive error in this example is simple myopia (SM).

EXAMPLE 2:
HIGH REFRACTIVE ERROR OF SIMPLE MYOPIA

Set the schematic eye to neutralization at the working distance, usually the zero setting (see Chapter 10, Practice Examples using Schematic Eye and Trial Lenses, p. 97, to properly set your schematic eye). Place a +5.50 sph in the slot closest to your schematic eye. This phantom lens is used to create the refractive error. Now, forget about the lens that was placed in the schematic eye and begin your retinoscopy. Start by looking at the reflex in the plano mirror position. You will see AGAINST, but since this much AGAINST is hard to see, reverse the sleeve of your retinoscope to the concave mirror position and see WITH motion. This tells you that you were seeing AGAINST with the plano mirror. Remember, in this special case of reversing the sleeve to the concave mirror position, if you see WITH motion, you will add *minus* lenses. This will then neutralize with a –5.50 sph.

EXAMPLE 3:
SIMPLE MYOPIC ASTIGMATISM

Place a +3.00 cylinder x 90° in the slot of your neutralized schematic eye. Begin your retinoscopy by establishing your two principle meridians. This will be 90° and 180°. With your retinoscopy in the plano mirror position you will see AGAINST at the 90° and no motion or neutral at 180°. If you can't see the AGAINST at 90°, reverse the sleeve of your retinoscope to the concave mirror position and see WITH.

If working in minus cylinder, neutralize the 180° meridian first. This will neutralize with a plano lens. Do your three tests to verify neutralization (p. 96) before proceeding to the second meridian at 90°. At the 90° meridian, you should see AGAINST motion (plano mirror position). If hard to see the AGAINST, reverse the sleeve of the retinoscope to the concave mirror position and see WITH. Add minus cylinder at the 90° meridian until neutralized. This will neutralize with a –3.00 cylinder x 90°. The final result will be: plano –3.00 x 90°.

If working in plus cylinder, the AGAINST motion at 90° might be hard to see in the plano mirror position, therefore reverse the sleeve of the retinoscope to the concave mirror position and see WITH motion. For WITH motion in the concave mirror position, add *minus* sphere. This will neutralize with a –3.00 sph. Do your three tests to verify neutral before proceeding to the 180° meridian. At the 180° meridian, you will see WITH motion in the plano mirror position. Add + cylinder at the 180° meridian until neutralized. This meridian will neutralize with a +3.00 cylinder x 180°. The final result will be: –3.00 + 3.00 x 180°.

EXAMPLE 4:
COMPOUND MYOPIC ASTIGMATISM

Place a +1.50 + 1.50 x 90° in the slots of your neutralized schematic eye. Begin your retinoscopy by establishing your two principle meridians. There will be AGAINST motion at the 90° and 180°. Again, if you have a hard time seeing the AGAINST motion, simply reverse the sleeve of your retinoscope to the concave mirror position. If you see WITH motion, add minus to neutralize in this concave mirror position.

If working in minus cylinder, neutralize the 180° meridian first. If you have a hard time seeing the AGAINST in the plano mirror position, simply reverse the sleeve of the retinoscope to the concave mirror position and see WITH. Then add *minus* sphere until neutralized with a –1.50 sph. Do your three tests to verify neutral at 180° before proceeding to the 90°. At the 90° meridian, you still see AGAINST in the plano mirror position, so reverse the sleeve to the concave mirror position and see WITH. Add minus cylinder until neutralized (–1.50 x 90°). The final result will be: –1.50 – 1.50 x 90°.

If working in plus cylinder, neutralize the 90° meridian first. At 90° see AGAINST in the plano mirror position, or reverse the sleeve of the retinoscope to the concave mirror position and see WITH. Then add *minus* in this concave mirror position. This will neutralize with a –3.00 sph. Do your three tests to verify neutral before proceeding to the 180° meridian. At the 180° meridian you will see WITH motion in the plano mirror position.

Add plus cylinder at the 180° meridian until neutralized (+1.50 x 180°). The final result will be −3.00 + 1.50 x 180°.

In all these examples, remember when working with plano mirror positions, if we see WITH we add plus, and for AGAINST we add minus. However, we do the *opposite* when working in the concave mirror position: seeing WITH we add minus and seeing AGAINST we add plus. If the reflex is neutral in the plano mirror position, it will also be neutral in the concave mirror position.

RETINOSCOPY AFTER REFRACTIVE SURGERY

Ron Stone, CRA

"Success is never final."
Winston Churchill

Retinoscopy has changed very little since its inception. However, the advances in corneal refractive surgery present us with new reflexes seen postoperatively. The need for possible new techniques causes us to re-evaluate our present abilities and retinoscopy routine. Retinoscopic reflexes after refractive surgery can be very misleading, depending on the procedure, patient, and post-operative complications. We have seen this in the past with RK and PRK, and even with PK (penetrating keratoplasty) procedures.

LASIK surgery presents its own set of unique reflexes. Differences in surgical techniques and instruments, lasers, surgeons, and patient corneas produce varied outcomes and results. The optical zone of the lasered area varies in size and geographic location on the cornea, as does the flap position and adhesion. To further complicate matters, the placement of the optical zone may not align with the patient's visual axis. All these variables blend together to give us a myriad of possible reflexes.

During the early postoperative period, especially the first week, these variables are fluctuating throughout each day, and from one day to the next. This makes our job as refractometrists much more exciting and frustrating at the same time. We need to be constantly aware of which procedure was performed for the patient. Our discussion here will be limited to LASIK, but the principle will apply to any postoperative cornea.

On the first few days postoperatively, we may not have a good retinoscopic reflex of any kind, nor any directional indications. Moving forward or rearward may prove valueless. Frequently, we may see two or three distinct areas for our reflex—which one we use is the ultimate question. We can be fooled if not paying close attention.

As you know, when in doubt you must concentrate on the reflex in the center of the pupil. This principle is particularly important after corneal surgery. As you approach neutralization in the center, you may be confused by seeing WITH or AGAINST reflexes appearing in the surrounding cornea. Be sure to watch closely for the point of neutralization (neutrality reflex). If you go too far, you may see an odd reflex, different from "scissors," wherein the reflex becomes wider in one meridian and narrower in the other. This appears to some as a "guillotine effect." So watch the center and judge NEUT when you still have a little WITH motion.

The first 30 days following laser procedures prove to be the most frustrating. Remain calm, since the situation is usually temporary. As edema subsides, the reflexes become sharper and easier to interpret. Just be sure to concentrate on the central portion and the treated areas of the cornea. Ignore the

Figure 12-1. Refractor reflections (lens is cross hatched). (A) Glare seen when you are centered on the axis. (B) The high reflex on the lens indicates that you are too high. (C) Ideal situation in which reflex is beside pupil. Purkinje images are visible in the center (the size of the reflexes has been reduced for clarity).

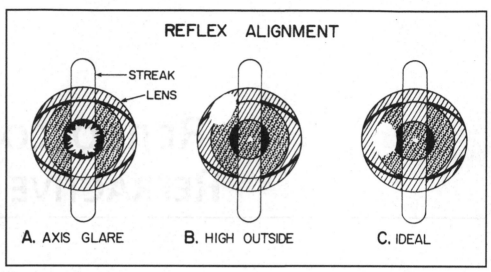

reflexes that vary considerably in the peripheral rim of the cornea. Do not be confused by these extra or contra-movements. Focus only on the central area.

Another occasional difficulty is surface reflections from the flat treated area, which interfere with interpreting the fundus reflex. When this is troublesome, simply move sideways to decenter these reflections off the pupil (Figure 12-1).

The main point is to concentrate solely on the central treated area. Do not be tricked by reflexes from the outer rim. Finally, be patient. This will become easier as the cornea heals and your skills improve. Good luck!

13

INTRODUCTION TO REFRACTION

*"Too often, patients dread this ordeal.
Relax, keep it simple, and be kind: accuracy will be your reward."*

Jay M. Enoch, PhD

By "refraction" (refractometry) we are referring to the process of both objective measurement (retinoscopy) and subjective verification.

Now that you grasp the essentials of retinoscopy, you can start using what you have learned. First, we will present some guidelines for smoothing the awkward transition from schematic eyes to refracting machines. Then, going beyond retinoscopy, we will consider how to test the patient's acceptance of your findings.

CLINICAL RETINOSCOPY

Retinoscopy provides a starting point for subjective testing, but now instead of placing lenses by hand, we will use a refracting machine.

The Refractor

You will ordinarily perform retinoscopy with a refractor (or Phoropter*). This machine contains all the lenses and accessories from the trial case (see Figure 5-5), arranged in discs, which can be rotated before the patient's eyes. A spring-balanced adjustable arm suspends the machine in front of the patient, who keeps his or her forehead in contact with the adjustable brow rest.

A refractor has three groups of discs, one each for spheres, cylinders, and accessories (including an occluder and +1.50 working lens). The lenses are arranged in 0.25 D increments, with spheres ranging from about −19.0 to +17.0 and cylinders to 6.0 D (plus *or* minus). We make strong sphere changes with the ±3.0 D auxiliary wheel. With a flick of the wrist, we can swing cross cylinders into place (as you will see on page 114), suspend a reading card, and adjust interpupillary distance (PD) and leveling. The vertex distance (VD) from the rear-most lens to the cornea may also be adjusted (within limits); the lens discs are vertex-compensated for their individual distances.

Most retinoscopists prefer plus cylinder refractors, for obvious reasons. If you do not have access to one, guidelines for retinoscopy with minus cylinder refractors are provided at the end of this chapter. Before you begin, be sure you are familiar with the controls on your retractor; this will spare you a lot of embarrassment (Figure 13-1). The large wheel on the outer edge of both sides controls the sphere power; rotate this *down* to move in a plus direction and up to move in a minus direction. Cylinder controls (for power and axis) are located near the center. The powers appear in windows near the controls, with black signifying plus and red signifying minus.

*This registered trademark for the American Optical refractor has crept into the language (along with Kleenex and Jello) as a generic term, referring to refracting machines in general.

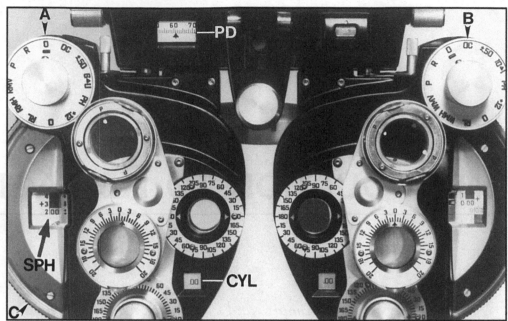

Figure 13-1. Phoropter, examiner's view. Right eye auxiliary dial (A) set at O indicates open aperture. Left eye dial (B) on OC shows aperture is closed. Sphere control for the right eye (C) has been set for +2.00 (SPH); the cylinder power (CYL) is zero. If these (cyl) numbers are black, this is a plus cyl phoropter; if red, this is a minus cyl instrument. Interpupillary distance (PD) and level adjustments are at top (courtesy of American Optical Co).

Your refractor permits greater accuracy by reducing patient fatigue and discomfort, but it makes measuring and controlling VD a difficult job. While you cannot retinoscope young children and certain disabled persons with a refractor, you will use it whenever possible. We reserve the trial frame (see Figure 13-7 on page 112) for confirming strong prescriptions (for example in aphakia where VD measurement is critical) and for testing acceptance of unusual prescriptions (oblique or unaccustomed cylinders, anisometropia, prisms, etc), but usually *not* for refracting.

Seat the patient comfortably in the examining chair, with his or her eyes on a level with yours. Clear the refractor by turning all the powers to zero, then swing it into position so you can see the patient's eyes through the open apertures, with the brow piece against his or her forehead. Adjust the brow rest for minimum VD, consistent with the length of the eyelashes, which may just touch the instrument but should not reach inside, or they will be snagged when you rotate the lenses.

Adjust the PD of the machine to the patient's distance PD (or at least be sure the corneal reflexes are centered in the apertures). Check the level and lock the arm.

Fixation and Fogging

In order to keep his or her eyes still and accommodation relaxed, your patient needs something to look at during retinoscopy. Ordinarily the patient fixes on a distant, *nonaccommodative* target, that is, any easily visible object without fine detail (which stimulates accommodation). A light usually provides the most suitable fixation device under the customary low illumination. Use a muscle light (if not too small), commercial device, or, if nothing else is available, the projected letter E (20/400 size). Dave Norath, COT, uses the projected red-green filter light without letters. This good nonaccommodative target eliminates the white-light reflections, which may confuse beginners.

The patient views the target at optical infinity (6 meters or 20 feet) either directly or with mirrors, which assures that the arriving wave front will be plano (see Figure 3-1C). We ask the patient to relax his eyes and gaze at the target. To further discourage accommodation, we may place a *fogging lens* before the fixing eye. "Fog" refers to the blurred image perceived when incoming rays focus *in front* of the retina. We create fog by adding positive vergence (plus power) to converge the incoming rays. For example,

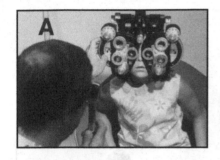

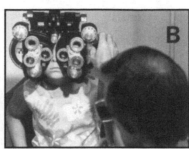

Figure 13-2. Ambidextrous retinoscopy. (A) Right eye: hold the scope in your right hand before your right eye. Left arm measures distance and changes lenses. (B) Left eye: all positions are reversed.

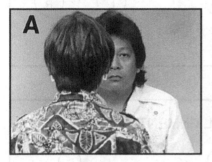

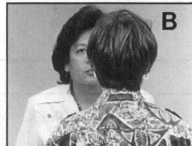

Figure 13-3. Refractor removed to show alignment. (A) Retinoscopy, right eye: patient maintains fixation with left eye gazing alongside examiner's right ear. (B) Retinoscopy, left eye: patient fixes with right eye. Note that examiner sits just enough to the side to avoid blocking patient's fixation.

if the patient were emmetropic, +2.0 sphere would produce a 2.0 D fog for distance objects (the image focuses 2.0 D in front of the retina). Similarly, a 2.0 D myope would be equally fogged for distance with a plano lens. (Do you understand why?)

The eye cannot clear the fogged image by accommodating, which in fact moves the focus further forward and increases the blur. Only by relaxed accommodation can the eye obtain the clearest image. A +1.50 D fogging lens reduces vision to about 20/100 or 20/200, making this a good choice.

Since we usually scope the right eye first, we will fog the left (fixing) eye about 1.50 D. If you know the previous distance correction, add approximately +1.50 D and place this power before the left eye (eg, if the patient wears +2.0, put up +3.50). If you do not know the prescription, just guess; if the patient has never worn a distance correction, start with +1.50. Turn the left sphere wheel until this power appears in the window, while advising the patient that this will make the target appear blurred.

Positioning and Alignment

While seated slightly to the patient's right, scope the right eye with your right eye. Your left arm measures the working distance and twirls the lenses

(Figure 13-2). The patient fixes the blurry target with her left eye.

When the patient's left (fixing) gaze passes just beside your right ear, you will be properly aligned (horizontally *and* vertically) for retinoscopy of the right eye. Reverse the positions when you move over to scope the left eye (Figure 13-3).

You must develop the ability to retinoscope with either eye (unless you have an amblyopia or other handicap), for only in this way can you maintain alignment while handling the scope and refractor, without breaking the patient's fixation. Look at this from above (Figure 13-4).

Note that when you finish scoping the right eye, the patient views the target through the gross retinoscopy lens, which normally fogs about 1.50 D. We will put this fog to advantage later when we come to subjective testing.

And when you now move to scope the left eye, the previous +1.50 D fogging lens becomes your working lens.

Optical Alignment

Students find retinoscopy with refractors difficult partly because of reflections from the lenses. Consequently, beginners unconsciously move too far laterally to avoid these reflexes. Actually, you

Figure 13-4. Positioning (overhead view). (A) Examiner scopes right eye with his; patient fixes distant target through fogging lens, left eye. (B) Examiner moves to patient's left to scope left eye with his; patient fixes through gross retinoscopy lens, right eye.

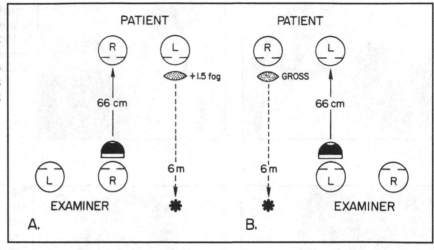

Figure 13-5. Refractor reflections (lens is cross hatched). (A) Glare seen when you are centered on the axis. (B) The high reflex on the lens indicates that you are too high. (C) Ideal situation when reflex is beside pupil. Purkinje images are visible in the center (the size of the reflexes has been reduced for clarity).

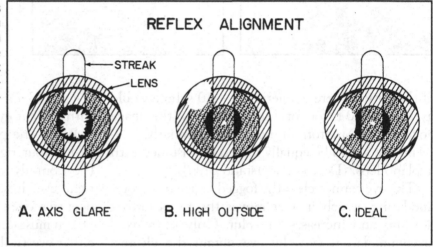

should see the reflections, but should displace them from the center of the lens by shifting your position slightly. Since the refractor lenses often obscure the Purkinje images (see Figure 5-7A), use these lens reflections to assist your alignment. The lens reflex should lie between the pupil and the lateral edge of the lens (Figure 13-5).

Retinoscopy

So now you have aligned everything and are ready to scope the right eye. Turn on the fixation light and retinoscope and turn off the room lights. Always keep a refracting lamp or nightlight on; never work in total darkness. It is difficult, clumsy, and possibly hazardous.

Scope the right eye just as you have learned, without the working lens (it just gets dirty and adds two reflecting surfaces). Survey the reflex. Get WITH in all meridians: spheric or astigmatic?

Neutralize the sphere, then determine cylinder axis and power. Recheck meridians and refine the sphere at working distance. When you are done, this gross serves as the fogging lens.

Move to the left eye and begin again, while the right eye fixes. When you finish the left, both eyes are fogged about 1.5 D. Calculate the net and record this for later self-analysis.

With experience you will require less than a minute or two to reach this point, that is, to retinoscope both eyes and record your findings. Now you are ready for the acid test.

SUBJECTIVE TESTING

In the *subjective* examination, you ask the patient what lenses help him to see best. You leave the optical science behind and begin a new ball game, involving quality of retinal images, integrity of the photoreceptors, neural pathways to the hindbrain, and responses of the occipital cortex. Integrative circuits analyze the stimulus and orchestrate a response, via subcortical relays, to a host of end organs that harmonize in reply, "Better."

We are dealing with the whole patient now, wherein intelligence, emotion, fatigue, and conditioning all play roles separate from the detection and perception of visual stimuli. Insofar as possible, you must reduce the interference these other factors impose. Put the patient at ease and gain his or her cooperation by using simple questions to frame easy choices. You will find it helpful to preface your tests by explaining that you only wish to know what the patient prefers and that, since "there is no right or wrong answer," the patient "cannot make a mistake."

Patients universally experience anxiety over the testing process, sometimes for very good reasons. Some impatient and less than sensitive examiners conduct refractions too quickly. Patients want to cooperate and respond appropriately, but the decisions are often very difficult; badgering patients throws them further into confusion (and sometimes panic or hostility), virtually guaranteeing invalid responses. Make it a point to have an annual refraction done by an inpatient colleague to maintain your empathy.

We *refine* the refraction in the same order as we performed retinoscopy; first the sphere, then cylinder axis and power. *We seek the stronger plus lens (or the weakest minus lens) that enables the patient to see best.* I prefer the patient to look at the projected letter chart showing five lines, from 20/50 at the top, to 20/20 at the bottom.

Refining the Sphere

We usually test the right eye first, although if you suspect unequal acuity (from the history or pre-refraction vision) always begin with the *better* eye.

Since the patient views the chart through the retinoscopy gross, he should be fogged (over-plussed) about 1.5 D. If your work has been reasonably accurate, *reducing* the sphere power six clicks (0.25 D each) should shift the image back to the retina. In practice you will be more accurate if you do this in steps, while at the same time *demonstrating* what you mean by "blurred" or "better." This

creates a kind of game that both reinforces and encourages the patient, while alleviating some of his or her fear of making an incorrect decision (and having to buy the wrong glasses). In Appendix I, you will find an example of such a testing "game" with the words I usually use.

You can save time if you avoid asking the patient what he or she sees or can read until you truly need that information. During sphere testing, you want only to know whether a lens is "better" or "no better."

As you reduce the fog in steps, the patient should see better with each lens. The endpoint is "no better." As your retinoscopy improves, you will find that the patient's choice of sphere usually agrees with yours, that is, the endpoint coincides with the lifting of the last trace of fog. When the patient does not agree with your findings, you may safely assume that you are wrong. Give the patient the sphere he wants (providing he sees better with it), and later, note how you differed; did you scope too much plus or too little minus?

Your patients are your instructors in refraction, so pay them heed and be a little humble.

Refining the Cylinder

We refine the astigmatic correction using Dr. Jackson's wondrous cross cylinder: a spherocylindric lens that has minus power in one meridian and plus power in the other. We use the cross cylinder (usually +0.25/–0.25 or +0.50/–0.50) to refine both the axis and power of the correcting cylinder. The crossed axes (Figure 13-6) lie 45° off the alignment of the handle (or the knurled knob, in the case of refractors, as you will see on p. 115) The plus meridian is marked with white dots, the minus, by red dots.

We flip the cylinder by rotating the handle, to show the patient two (blurred) images, and we ask him to compare the blur. The endpoint with cross cylinder testing is "equally bad."

First, we test for axis: we align the cross cylinder handle with the astigmatic axis, so that the plus meridian lies 45° off to one side (Figure 13-6A1). Then we rotate the handle, flipping the plus meridian to the other side of the axis (Figure 13-6A2). The patient compares the two images to see if either of them appears less blurred. If one position

Figure 13-6. Confirming the cylinder. For axis (A.1, A.2) align the handle with axis of the correcting cylinder. Flip plus meridian 45° to each side. For power (B.1, B.2) place the handle 45° off the cylinder axis. Flip plus and minus meridians into alignment, changing cylinder power according to better position.

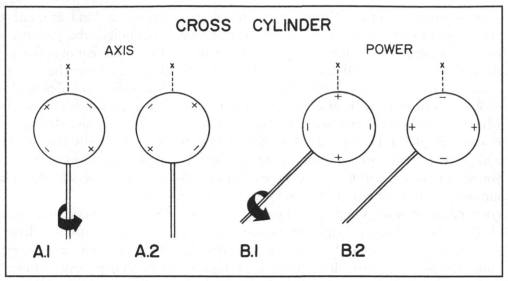

of the plus meridian appears clearer, turn the correcting plus cylinder in that direction. (When using minus cylinders, we turn the correcting minus cylinder toward the clearer position of the minus meridian). Then realign the handle with this new axis and repeat the test. (How far you initially turn the correcting cylinder depends on the patient's response and the size of the cylinder; perhaps 10° for a 1.0 D cylinder, proportionately less in high powers. Make smaller changes as you near the endpoint.) When both positions are equally blurred, you move on to refining the cylinder power. When in doubt, favor the patient's accustomed axis.

Next, we test for power: we turn the handle so it lies 45° off the axis of astigmatism. As we flip the lens, we alternately align the plus and minus meridians with the axis of the correcting cylinder. When we place the plus meridian over the axis (Figure 13-6B.1), we increase the cylinder power. When we place the minus meridian over the cylinder, we reduce its power (Figure 13-6B.2). We change the power of the correcting cylinder according to the patient's preference. In other words, if the image appears better with the minus meridian over the axis, we reduce the cylinder power; if the image improves with the plus meridian aligned, we increase the power. The endpoint is "equally bad." When in doubt, give less cylinder power.

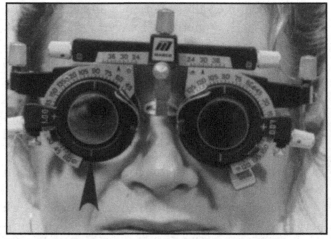

Figure 13-7. Before refining the cylinder, a patient wears plano +1.00 x 90, in this trial frame.

THE CLINICAL SEQUENCE

Let's look at how a typical cross cylinder sequence might proceed. We will use a trial frame in these illustrations for clarity. Let's say that after you have refined the sphere, the patient wears plano +1.00 x 90 in each eye. You occlude the left eye (Figure 13-7).

To refine the axis, we align the cross cylinder handle with the correcting cylinder axis. We flip the plus meridian from one side to the other, asking the patient which position is better (Figure 13-8A).

The patient prefers position two (Figure 13-8B), so we rotate the cylinder axis toward the white dots,

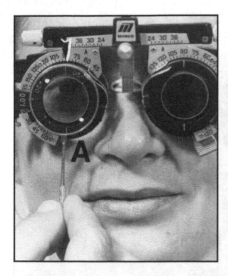 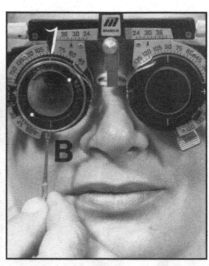

Figure 13-8. Axis test: handle on axis at 90. (A) White dots (plus) lie to one side of the axis. (B) Lens has been flipped and dots now lie on the other side.

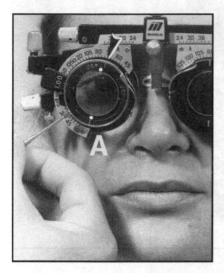 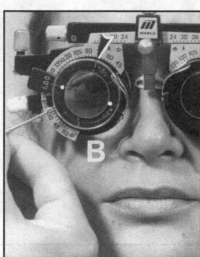

Figure 13-9. Power test: handle 45° off axis 80. (A) White dots are on axis, increasing plus power (B) Lens is flipped and white dots are off axis (red dots, minus, are on), reducing plus power.

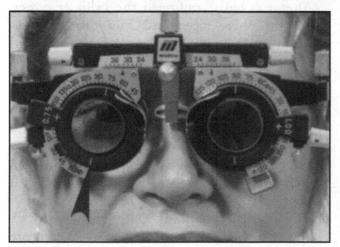

Figure 13-10. After refining the cylinder, the patient wears plano +0.75 x 80.

that is, clockwise to 80°. We repeat the test and now she says, "both equally bad." This means he or she prefers the axis at 80°, so we now have plano +1.00 x 80.

Now we test for *power* by turning the cross cylinder handle 45° off this axis. We place the plus meridian on axis 80, then flip it off, asking which position is better (Figure 13-9A).

Our patient prefers position two (Figure 13-9B), the position of less plus. We reduce the cylinder power 0.25 (to +0.75), and repeat the test. He or she now says, "equally blurred." So we stop here.

The patient has rotated our cylinder axis 10° and reduced its power by 0.25 D (Figure 13-10). We give the lens he or she has chosen because the patient, like the customer, is always right. Usually.

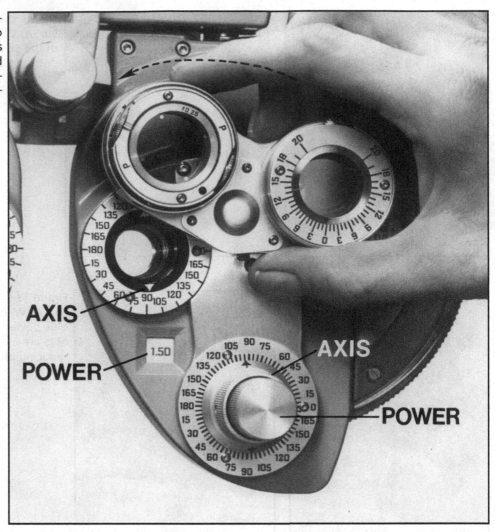

Figure 13-11. Rotating the turret to bring cross cylinder into position. The concentric knobs (below) control axis and power of the correcting cylinder; power shows in the window beneath the aperture.

Figures 13-11 through 13-14 demonstrate the use of the cross cylinder on the refractor (courtesy of American Optical Co).

The way we do this cylinder testing is shown in Appendix I, Act II.

There is an additional concept called the "*spherical equivalent*"[1] that you will need for refining cylinder power. This refers to the *dioptric midpoint* of the astigmatic images which changes when you alter the cylinder power. To maintain spherical equivalence, you compensate the sphere when changing the power of the cylinder. If you alter the cylinder power more than 0.50 D, you adjust the sphere by *half* this amount in the *opposite* direction in order to keep the cross cylinder images straddling the retina. For example, if you *reduce* the plus cylinder 0.50 D, you *increase* the sphere +0.25 D before repeating the power test.

After you have confirmed the cylinder power, *recheck* the sphere once again. Only at this point do you need to inquire what the patient sees; record the vision while he reads.

Now you occlude the right eye, and repeat the entire process with the left eye.

Binocular Balance

You have now measured the best vision in each eye separately; *if they are roughly equal*, you may wish to confirm your endpoints by *balancing* the vision under binocular conditions. Place a light fog (0.75 D) before both eyes and ask the patient to compare the blurred letters as you alternately occlude each eye. Give the better eye 0.25 D more fog, then compare again. The endpoint is: "Equally bad." If the fog reverses the "better" eye, leave the dominant eye seeing best. Usually, both eyes will balance

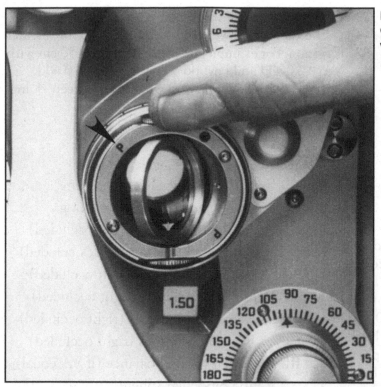

Figure 13-12. Flipping cross cylinder for axis test. Cross cylinder "handle" (thumb knob) aligned with axis. Note P (power) 45° off axis.

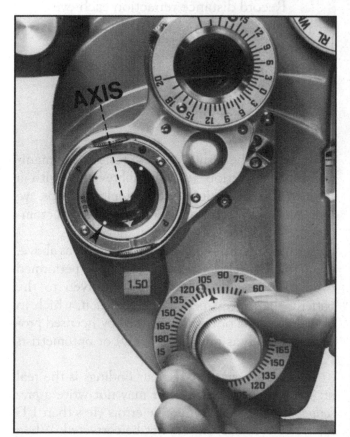

Figure 13-13. Adjusting the axis. Knob controls axis of the correcting cylinder; the cross cylinder automatically rotates along with the cylinder axis.

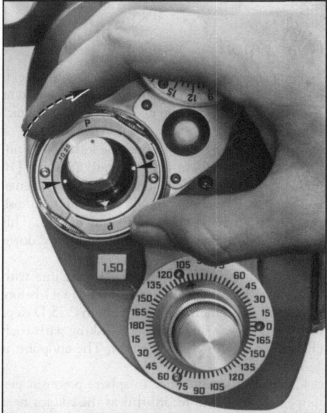

Figure 13-14. Rotating cross cylinder "handle" into position for power test. Knob now lies 45° off axis, while red/white (power) dots are on axis.

Table 13-1

Add for Age: Average Additional Sphere Required by Emmetropes for Reading at 40 cm	
Age	*Add*
45	+0.75
50	+1.25
55	+1.75
60	+2.00
65	+2.25
70	+2.50

within 0.25 D. Obviously, this will be misleading if an eye is amblyopic or diseased; never sacrifice acuity for the sake of balance.

When you reduce the binocular balancing fog in steps, you may find that the patient accepts 0.25 D more plus under these conditions; frequently the *duochrome test*[2] helps to refine the binocular sphere. The patient will now usually read one line better than under monocular conditions.

In Act III of Appendix I, we show how to say this.

Near Vision

The patient is now fully corrected for distance. If he or she is over 40, hyperopic, or has symptoms related to near vision, you need to check the refraction at *near*.

Turn the room lights on and the letter chart off. Lower the reading arm with the card at 40 cm (16 inches), the best distance for testing most patients. Converge the refractor (or adjust the PD) and ask the patient to read the lowest line he can. This stimulates accommodation while you copy down the *distance* lens powers from the refractor.

If the patient cannot read the lowest line with ease, place half the *add for age* (Table 13-1) before *both* eyes. Then increase the sphere in 0.25 D steps before both eyes simultaneously, asking with each click whether the vision is better. The endpoint is "no better."

Calculate the difference in sphere power at distance and near, and record this as the *add* for near (eg, if the distance sphere is +0.50, and the near is +2.0, the add is +1.50—see Appendix I, Act IV).

Avoid giving more add than necessary because the dioptric power limits the far point of distinct vision. For example, images blur beyond 50 cm with a +2.0 add and beyond 33 cm with a +3.0 add.

Here is a summary of what you've been doing. Keep it handy.

Refraction Flow Sheet:
  I. Retinoscopy right eye (left fixing)
     Retinoscopy left eye (right fixing)
 II. A. Refine right sphere (left occluded)
        Refine right cylinder (left occluded)
        Record right vision (left occluded)
     B. Refine left sphere (right occluded)
        Refine left cylinder (right occluded)
        Record left vision (right occluded)
III. Binocular fog and balance (if VA equal)
     Refine binocular sphere
     Record distance refraction each eye
 IV. Binocular add for near
     Record add

The Prescription

We record the results of these tests as the manifest (dry) refraction (usually abbreviated with a large M). If the patient had cycloplegic drops, we indicate this by a large C). Compare this refractometry with your retinoscopy.

Retinoscopy and subjective refinement, as above, are defined as *refractometry*, and may be performed by technicians. If a prescription is given to the patient, the process becomes a *refraction*, which in most states may only be performed by licensed professionals such as physicians (MD) or optometrists (OD).

What you now do with your findings is the real art of refracting. You may or may not write a *prescription*. Most small refractive errors (less than 1 D sphere or cylinder) should not be corrected. When you do write a prescription, you will usually modify the results of your refraction, depending on the patient's symptoms, previous prescriptions and type of glasses, muscle balance, occupation, etc.

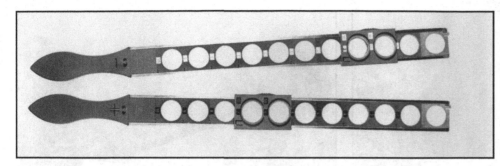

Figure 13-15. Retinoscopy (skiascopy) racks; minus above and plus below. Each has ten spheres (1.0 to 10.0 D), plus sliding auxiliaries (0.50 and 10.0 D). This provides a range from plano to 10.50 in 0.50 D steps and from 11.0 to 20.0 in 1.0 D steps (Western Ophthalmics, WO-180).

Because it is "difficult to improve on satisfaction," beware prescribing simply because you have discovered a refractive error. The cost of glasses is more than money, and prescribing unnecessarily will harm you, if not the patient.

Keep foremost in mind that we prescribe glasses for only three reasons: 1) to help the patient *see* better (if that is his or her desire); 2) to help the patient *feel* better (if the prescription will likely relieve the symptoms); and 3) to help the patient *look* better (if the glasses correct strabismus, mask ptosis, etc). Only if you can reasonably expect the prescription to fulfill one of these criteria, may you prescribe with confidence that your efforts will be appreciated.

Golden Rules

Do not prescribe glasses unless necessary (see above); do not change a lens unless vision or symptoms will significantly improve; and do not make too great a change (more than one diopter) at once.

Subjective Summary

You will develop your own methods for subjective testing, and in time you will find the words to communicate best with different types of patients. Not knowing what to say or do in an organized sequence presents a big obstacle in the beginning. In Appendix I, you will find my simple refraction routine, which may prove helpful to you.

Remember this paradox: the more time you spend on the subjective examination, the less accurate it becomes. Keep it short and keep it simple. Put the patient at ease and remind him that he cannot make a mistake. Be sure to cultivate equanimity; you can't get a 20/20 refraction from a 20/200 brain.

SPECIAL CIRCUMSTANCES

Cycloplegia

We usually perform retinoscopy with an undilated pupil to avoid spherical aberration and irregular reflexes. If active accommodation forces you to use cycloplegic drops (in children or hyperopes), be sure to watch the pupil center to avoid edge reflexes. Since the drops relax accommodation, you may improve alignment by having the patient fix on the scope or on your ear, or you may use an interesting near target to improve fixation. Young hyperopes will accept more plus under cycloplegia; a lens thus prescribed will usually blur the vision when the drops wear off. We usually recheck the refraction at a later date (so-called *postcheck*) to be sure of the patient's acceptance under more physiologic circumstances.

Portable Retinoscopy

Whether you retinoscope aphakic or strabismic infants in the operating room or geriatric patients in a nursing home, *skiascopy* racks (Figure 13-15) prove very convenient. You may carry a pair in your pocket to avoid hauling the trial case along. With lens racks we use the spheres method, described on page 64. When we have no refractor but require greater accuracy than the spheres method allows, we retinoscope over the patient's glasses, especially with strong corrections (eg, in aphakic persons) using *Halberg clips* (seen on the patient in Figure 13-23).

For measuring strong plus corrections under anesthesia (infants after congenial cataract aspiration may require +23.0 D or more), Enoch has devised a simple, accurate retinoscopy method based on vertex distances.[3]

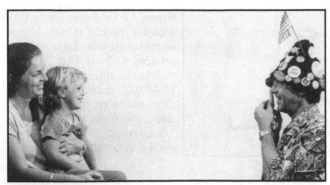

Figure 13-16. Survey the reflex. Keep your distance while you make friends; if necessary, neutralize at one meter. Toys and silly hats help to put the child at ease.

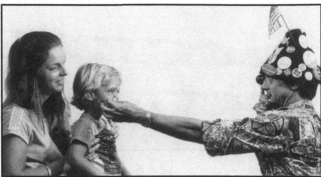

Figure 13-17 Hand-held lens. If the child is wary, use hand-held lenses. Hold the fixation target in your teeth.

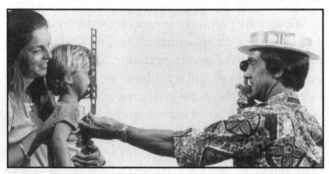

Figure 13-18. Lens rack. This proves priceless for quick neutralizing. Some children mistake it for a paddle, so present it carefully.

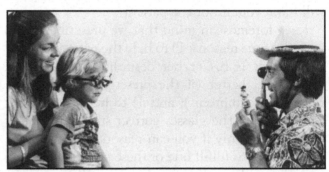

Figure 13-19. Child trial frame. Most youngsters will accept this comfortable, lightweight device. We usually use this for large cylinders, which demand real accuracy (straddling).

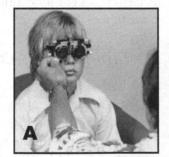 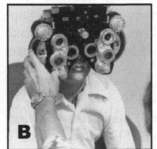

Figure 13-20. Do not use a trial frame (A) after age six. Many modern youngsters enjoy the refractor (B), especially when we liken it to an "astronaut's binocular" or "space scanner."

Retinoscopy with Children

Most of us do poorly with children. Their unpredictability and lack of cooperation threaten our composure; once a child starts to scream, retinoscopy comes to a halt. We are powerless against closed lids and force makes matters worse (Figures 13-16 through 13-22).

Success in retinoscopy of children lies in *prevention*. Treat children with respect because, like grenades, they're explosive. Keep your distance and do not get too cozy until you have "made friends." Move slowly, make reassuring sounds, and have lots of interesting, noisy toys. Tell the child what you are going to do, and first demonstrate retinoscopy (or eye drops, etc) on a parent or yourself.

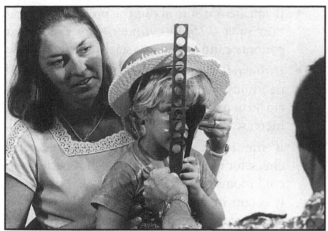

Figure 13-21. Strabismus. To maintain alignment when retinoscoping the deviating eye, the mother occludes the dominant eye.

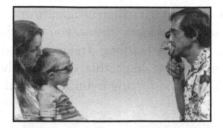

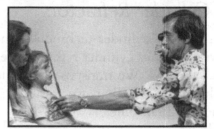

Figure 13-22. Off-axis. Child is too low, making alignment difficult (top). Child looks up through the edge of trial lens, disturbing the reflex (bottom).

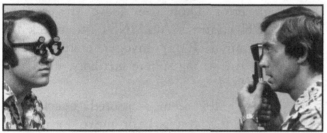

Figure 13-23. Halberg Clips. Retinoscopy over the patient's glasses. The clips hold the lenses.

Fixation

Children up to age 4 or 5 are more at ease sitting on the parent's lap. Since we usually employ cycloplegics, near-targets are acceptable; hold fixation toys in your free hand or teeth. Older children generally sit by themselves, with a parent seated at the end of the room. For fixation, the children can count his or her mother's fingers. Some refractionists use animated toys or even movies.

Remember that by using various estimating techniques, you can frequently learn all you need without lenses.

Retinoscopy of children can be trying. If you keep cool, it can be very satisfying; in time, you will be winning more than you lose. Copeland wrote an excellent article on this subject which you should review.[4]

OTHER TRICKS

Incident Neutral

The term "incident neutral" refers to the red reflex we produce by focusing the retinoscope beam on the retina (as opposed to emergent neutral, the reflex we see at NEUT).[5] From the working distance, you create incident neutral by lowering the sleeve a little beyond the midpoint (where the intercept focuses on the pupil), until you see the bright orange fundus glow. We use this reflex to study the media by retroillumination, usually with the pupil dilated. It is a great way to demonstrate cataract, vitreous floaters, or corneal opacities, which appear black against the red background. Try it on your partner.

Retinoscopy Over Glasses

By simply holding a working lens before the patient's glasses, you can check the prescription (see Figure 6-9). When the patient wears a very strong correction, you can save time and avoid VD problems by retinoscopy over his lenses using Halberg clips—miniature trial frames that snap on the glasses. This trick also proves helpful in nursing homes and other places where a refractor is not handy, because you can achieve greater accuracy than with lens racks using the spheres method (Figure 13-23).

When a patient with high astigmatism complains of distortion in his new glasses, you can check the cylinder axis by straddling (refer to Figure 8-9) through a working lens; this confirms the exact location of the correcting cylinder in front of the eye.

Minus Cylinder Refractors

To employ plus cylinder techniques when confronted with a minus cylinder refractor, we use the *double-click* method. We transpose the cylinder (p. 92) mechanically, so that we can use friendly WITH motion at all times.

Here's how:

1. Refine your sphere in the usual manner. When you are done, you will have residual WITH in the cylindric meridian.

2. Set the cylinder axis *perpendicular* to your cylindric meridian.

3. Neutralize the WITH reflex by using the controls for both cylinder and sphere: to create + 0.25 cylinder in the correct meridian, click 0.25 minus cylinder accompanied by 0.25 plus sphere.

Thus for each click (–0.25) of cylinder, you click (+0.25) the sphere. This transposes the cylindrical effect to that of a plus cylinder in the proper meridian. When using this double-click technique, refine cylinder axis and power by *minus* cylinder rules (p. 92). For subjective testing, the cross cylinder axis test follows the *red* (minus) dots; the power test follows logic.

The double-click method sounds complicated, but really becomes a simple reflex in a few minutes: you click (minus cylinder) and click (plus sphere) until you have neutralized the cylindric reflex. To prevent error, first record your refraction directly from the refractor and then transpose this to plus cylinder form.

MISCELLANEOUS TIPS

Here are some final thoughts on handling common difficulties:

- If you see the reflex changing, the patient is accommodating. If you cannot control this, quit and use cycloplegics.

- If you are not sure about the presence or location of a 0.25 D cylinder, forget it. Most patients cannot detect a small cylinder, anyway.

- If the reflex appears too dim, move in and neutralize at some closer point (perhaps 25 cm), then allow for the working distance, or increase the scope voltage or dilate the pupil.

- If the reflex disappears while you scope, check for fogging of the lens—hot patients in cold rooms can steam the lenses. This usually occurs in the morning, before the refractor has warmed up; increasing the VD a little usually helps.

- If the pupil is dilated, be sure to watch the center.

- If the reflex appears motionless, it is usually high error. Drop the sleeve (reversal to WITH confirms AGAINST) to check for high minus. If not myopia, crank in plus using the strong sphere auxiliary, until you see WITH.

- If the reflex seems scissored, check your alignment (off-axis?), or move in (was it merely AGAINST?). Try the direct retinoscopy method (p. 86), then use this estimate for subjective testing (avoiding neutralizing altogether). If all else fails, check the keratometer readings, and look for distortion of the mires (it may be keratoconus).

Once you are confident, you will find you can save time by setting the axis of the refractor cylinder at the same axis as the patient's glasses cylinder and by scoping the opposite (spheric) meridian first. Similarly, do not spend time refining a cylinder axis by retinoscopy, if the patient can manage this himself with the cross cylinder.

Remember that the most of the time we use retinoscopy to provide baseline measurements, so that the patient can more quickly refine the refraction. You do not ordinarily need to be very accurate, except when the patient cannot cooperate for subjective testing. We learn to improve our accuracy primarily so that we can help the 5% of patients who can't help themselves.

When refracting alert adults you will usually find you can best use your time by doing a quick "ballpark" retinoscopy, followed by more careful subjective refinement in the time saved.

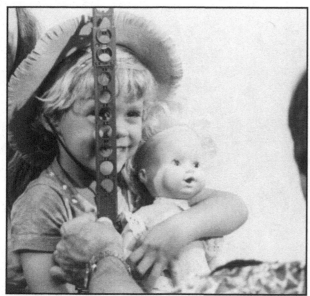

Figure 13-24. Smile. Have fun!

By continually comparing your retinoscopy with the manifest refraction, you will improve faster, and will learn to appraise your accuracy under various circumstances. By self-analysis you will develop confidence; that is, you will know when to trust your measurements, and when to rely on the patient.

In the meantime, have fun. And smile (Figure 13-24)!

The retinoscope is like a grand piano. Whether you never get beyond "Chopsticks," or progress to a Rachmaninoff Piano Concerto, is up to you.

"The only things worth learning, are the things you learn after you know it all."

Harry S. Truman

REFERENCES

1. Isenstein C. Clinical application of the conoid of Sturm. In Sloan AE, ed. *Manual of Refraction*. 2nd ed. Boston, Mass: Little, Brown and Co; 1970:73.

2. Michels DD. *Vision Optics and Refraction, A Clinical Approach*. St. Louis, Mo: CV Mosby; 1970:231,238.

3. Copeland JC. The refraction of children with special reference to retinoscopy. *Int Ophthalmol Clin*. 1970;3:959-970.

4. Enoch JM. A rapid, accurate technique for retinoscopy of the aphakic infant or child in the operating room. *Am J Ophthalmol*. 1974;78:335-336.

5. Pascal JI. The "incidence neutral" point in retinoscopy. *Arch Ophthalmol*. 1948;39:550-551.

APPENDIX I: SPEEDY REFRACTION

AN ORIGINAL PLAY IN FOUR ACTS FEATURING RETINOSCOPY, FOGGING, AND SUBJECTIVE

ACT I: RETINOSCOPY

Patient at refractor, both eyes open; no lens right, left eye fixes distant light through 1.50 D fogging lens.*

Doctor: "NOW JUST RELAX YOUR EYES AND LOOK AT THE BLURRED LIGHT." Scope his right eye, with your right eye (while he fixes with left). Move over to scope left eye (right eye now fixes through 1.50 D gross fog).

Doctor: "THE LIGHT IS STILL BLURRED. JUST RELAX AND WATCH IT." Scope left eye with your left eye (while he fixes with right). There is now 1.50 D fog before both eyes. Flip target light off, letter chart on (lines 20/50 to 20/20).

ACT II: FOGGING SUBJECTIVE

Scene One: Sphere

Occlude left (right is 1.50 D fogged).

Doctor: "NOW I'VE PUT SOME LETTERS UP THERE, BUT THEY ARE ALL BLURRED."

Patient: "LIKE, WOW!"

Doctor: "NOW I'M GOING TO MAKE THEM BETTER, A LITTLE AT A TIME." Rapidly unfog four clicks (now 0.50 D fog). "THAT'S BETTER, ISN'T IT?"

Patient: "FOR SURE!"

Unfog one click (now 0.25 D fog).

Doctor: "THAT'S *STILL* BETTER, RIGHT?"

Patient: "RIGHT."

Doctor: "NOW, IS THE NEXT ONE REALLY BETTER?"

Unfog one click (now about zero fog).

Patient: "YUP, BETTER."

Doctor: "GOOD. NOW IS THE NEXT ONE *REALLY* BETTER? OR ABOUT THE SAME?" ("SMALLER, BLACKER, FURTHER AWAY?")

Click one more (should be overminused).

Patient: "NOPE. NO BETTER."

Back up one lens. Stop there.

Scene Two: Cylinder

For cylinder axis (cross cylinder meridian 45° off cylinder axis):

Doctor: "HERE ARE TWO CHOICES (lenses):

---

*"Fogging lens" refers to a lens of increased vergence (plus) power. When we fog we increase the sphere (in a plus direction). We unfog by reducing the sphere (in minus direction).

THEY ARE BOTH BAD (blurred). SEE IF ONE OF THEM IS BETTER THAN THE OTHER."

"THIS IS THE FIRST (pause) AND (flip lens) THIS IS THE SECOND."

Refine axis, turning cylinder toward "better" position of white (plus) dots: endpoint is equal blur.

Doctor: "NOW ARE THEY ABOUT EQUALLY BAD?"

Patient: "YEAH, BOTH BAD."

For cylinder power (cross cylinder meridians aligned with cylinder axis).

Doctor: "NOW HERE ARE TWO MORE BAD CHOICES. SEE IF ONE OF THEM IS BETTER. THIS IS THE FIRST," (pause) "AND (flip lens) THIS IS THE SECOND."

Refine power, according to desire for more plus or less plus; endpoint is equal blur (in doubt, favor less power). Remove cross cylinder.

Finale

Doctor: "WHAT IS THE LOWEST LINE YOU CAN READ?"

Patient: "T... Z... V..."

Doctor: "GOOD!"

Recheck sphere power (especially if cylinder power was changed more than 0.50 D). Now, occlude right, open left. (Left is 1.50 D fogged.) Repeat entire act with left eye.

Act III: Balance

Now open right. Both are open with best distance correction.

Doctor: "NOW THAT'S VERY CLEAR WITH TWO EYES RIGHT?"

Patient: "RIGHT! WOW!"

From now on, change lenses simultaneously (with both hands, before both eyes).

Doctor: "I'M GOING TO MAKE IT WORSE NOW..."

Fog one click (0.25 D).

"AND WORSE..."

Fog another click (now 0.50 D).

"AND WORSE YET..."

Fog another (now 0.75 D).

"NOW, THAT'S VERY BLURRED, RIGHT?"

Patient: "HEY, WHAT'S HAPPENING?"

Use hand-held occluder to cover each eye alternately.

Doctor: "NOW, TELL ME, IS IT ABOUT EQUALLY BAD... RIGHT EYE? (shift cover) LEFT EYE?"

Repeat and balance by adding + 0.25 to "better" eye. Endpoint is equal blur.

Doctor: "NOW, WE'LL MAKE IT BETTER..."

Unfog both eyes one click (now 0.50 D fog).

"AND STILL BETTER...?"

Unfog one click (now 0.25 D fog).

"NOW IS THE NEXT ONE *REALLY* BETTER, OR ABOUT THE SAME?"

Unfog one click (now about zero fog). Push plus, if in doubt. Usually, accepts +0.25 D more under binocular conditions. Now balanced for distance, with maximum plus. May check binocular endpoint with duochrome.

Act IV: Near Subjective

This is done only after age 40 (30 if hyperopic), or if the patient has symptoms at near. Flip on room light, drop down the reading card at 16 inches and converge the refractor.

Doctor: "NOW, JUST LOOK AT THE CARD FOR A MOMENT." ("CAN YOU READ ANYTHING?")

Stimulates accommodation, while you copy down distance Rx to this point. (He has no add yet.)

Change lenses with both hands, simultaneously before both eyes. Now, click-in roughly half of "add for age" (p. 116).

Doctor: "NOW, THAT'S BETTER, RIGHT?"

Increase sphere in 0.25 D steps, following each with...

"IS THAT BETTER? ("IS IT *REALLY* BETTER?"), etc.

Endpoint is when it is not really better. This is important. Don't give too much add!

Doctor: "NOW READ THE BOTTOM LINE FOR ME."

While reading, you compute and record add.

End: Total time is 3 to 6 minutes.

Note: The program is short; there is less fatigue, more accuracy.

Patient is seldom asked to read.

You reinforce the patient and teach him what you mean, so the refraction becomes a game. Fogging and balancing are incorporated.

Critique: You cannot always give equal adds, especially in amblyopes with unequal accommodation, but these are rare.

Appendix II: Maintaining the Optec 360 Retinoscope

Ron Stone, CRA

As time goes by, fine dust and haze accumulate on the mirror of the retinoscope, as well as on the lens and bulb. This film reduces the brightness of the projected light beam entering the eye, thus dimming the emerging retinal reflex. In addition, the film obscures the aperture on the mirror, through which you are viewing this dimmer reflex. Thus, it becomes progressively more difficult to see what you are doing.

So periodically your scope should be cleaned to keep it (and you) operating at full capacity. Try it yourself. If you are reading this, then you have already shown an interest. You can do it.

We are about to tackle disassembling, cleaning, and reassembling of your Copeland-Optec 360 Streak retinoscope. We have chosen this popular model for our instructions, but the principles are similar with other scopes.

You will need a couple of tools and some supplies. Gather up a small eyeglass screwdriver with a standard tip, a medium standard screwdriver, and Phillips' screwdriver (some scopes have a mixture of screw heads, so use the appropriate match). You will also need a lens cloth (the satin-type for plastic spectacle lenses, not the paper type for camera lenses), a few alcohol preps, a couple of tissues, a cotton-tipped applicator, and a clean work space. Set aside about 45 minutes to an hour. Your speed will increase with practice.

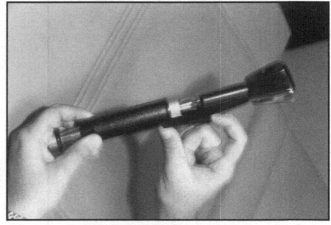

Figure A-1. Gently lifting thumb slide rest.

Now let's get started.

Disassembly

Step 1: Remove the battery/light housing unit by gently lifting up in the thumb slide rest. Slide the battery/light housing unit out the bottom of the handle (Figure A-1).

Step 2: Remove the two small screws on the aluminum face plate. Set them aside in a safe place where they will not be lost (Figure A-2).

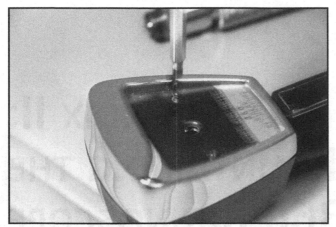

Figure A-2. Removing face plate screws.

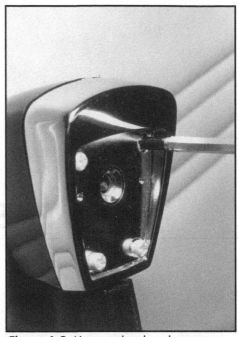

Figure A-3. Unscrewing head screws.

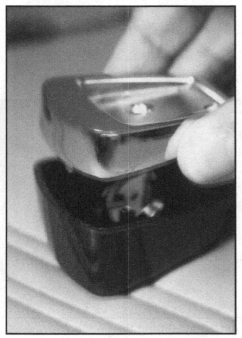

Figure A-4. Lifting and separating chrome head piece.

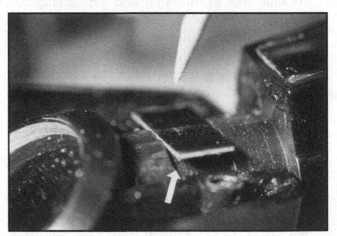

Figure A-5. Spring tensioner atop battery/light tube.

Step 3: Unscrew the four screws in the head unit. They may not come out all the way, but be sure they are all unscrewed fully (Figure A-3). Carefully lift and separate the chrome piece (Figure A-4).

Step 4: Look for the flat spring tensioner lying on top of the battery tube (Figure A-5). Set it aside with small screws from the face plate.

Step 5: Lift the battery/light tube from the plastic half of the head unit, being careful not to lose the lens from the top of the battery

tube (Figure A-6). Carefully tip the battery tube bottom up and allow the lens to fall into your hand (Figure A-7).

Step 6: Now the most important part, the mirror. Lift or drop out the mirror CAREFULLY (Figure A-8)! The mirror has both front and back mirrored surfaces. The front mirrored surface is down, or faces the patient (Figure A-9). The back surfaced mirror faces you. Can you tell the difference? Take any dull object and place it on the mirror. If the reflected image touches, it is front

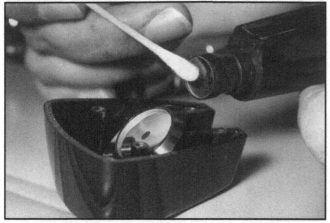

Figure A-6. Protecting lens atop battery/light tube.

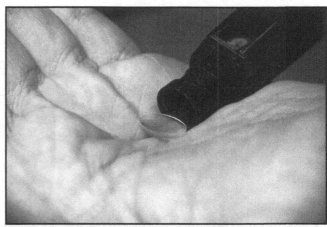

Figure A-7. Catching lens in your hand.

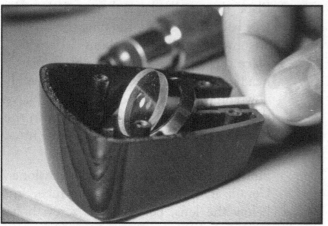

Figure A-8. Removing mirror.

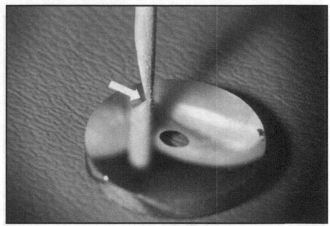

Figure A-9. Mirror front surface. Note images touch (arrow).

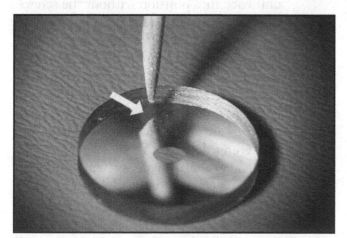

Figure A-10. Mirror back surface. Note images don't touch (arrow).

surfaced (faces patient). If there is a slight gap between the object and the reflection, it is the back surface (faces you) (Figure A-10). Magic!

Step 7: Clean all the parts. Using an alcohol prep, wipe down the black plastic and chrome half of the head unit, the battery/light tube, and the face plate. Use a fresh alcohol prep on the mirror for both sides, front-sided surface first, then back-sided surface. Use the lens cloth to gently wipe the surfaces dry. You can use the same prep for the battery/light tube lens. Wipe down the chrome battery/light housing and lamp. Make sure the illumination lamp is properly seated, without leaving your fingerprints on the bulb, and be certain that both ends of the housing are screwed in all the way.

OK, great, so far. Time to reassemble:

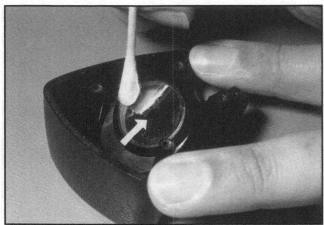

Figure A-11. Replacing mirror. Note "no touch" technique on front surface, oval window vertical (arrow).

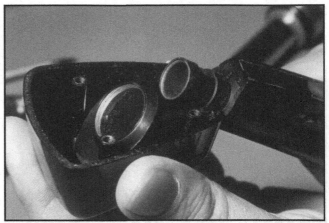

Figure A-12. Lens replaced in battery/light tube, and tube placed in head.

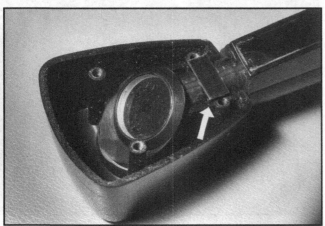

Figure A-13. Spring tensioner centered between screw holes.

Re-Assembly

Step 1: Place the mirror back into the black half of the head unit, face (front surface) down, with the back (glass surface) toward you. Be sure that you leave no fingerprints. You must make sure that the oval "window" in the center of the mirror is aligned straight up and down (Figure A-11). If it is not, do not remove the mirror to adjust its position. Instead, grab that cotton-tipped applicator and wipe it around the edges of the mirror. Make sure the back of the mirror toward you is the (glass) back surface. Using the wood side of the applicator, spin it around the entire mirror edge in either direction you need it to go to align the oval vertically.

Step 2: Place the small plastic battery/light tube lens back in position. Keeping the tube in an upward position at about 50° to 60°, place the tube back into the black plastic head unit (Figure A-12). Lay this assembly down on the work surface. You should have the mirror still in position, the lens in the battery/light tube, and the two units fitted together.

Step 3: Find the little flat metal spring tensioner. Center it on the battery/light tube, just below the lens, between the screw holes (Figure A-13).

Step 4: Gently place the chrome half of the head unit back into position without the screws. Once in position, place all 4 screws into the holes. DO NOT immediately screw them in. First, rotate each counter-clockwise, until the screw "drops" into position. You will feel it. Once the screw drops into position, screw it in halfway. Make sure all 4 screws are started and halfway in before tightening down on them (Figure A-14). Remember that you are screwing into plastic, which can strip or break easily. Seat the screws firmly—a "death grip" tightness is not needed.

Step 5: Replace the face plate with the 2 small screws. Tighten until they are firmly in position.

Step 6: Replace the battery housing into the retinoscope (Figure A-15).

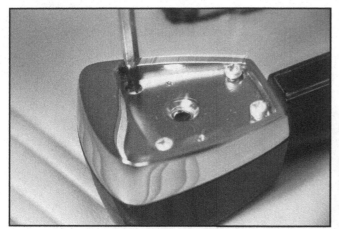

Figure A-14. Make sure all screws are started, before tightening any.

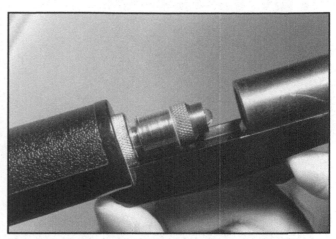

Figure A-15. Replacing battery housing with bulb.

Congratulations! You are now an official retinoscope maintenance technician! With a little more practice, you will be able to do this in no time at all. There is no need to call anyone to fix or service your retinoscopes. You can do it. You can be back in service much faster, and much more efficiently.

All figures courtesy of Andrew Yuen, BA, CRA.

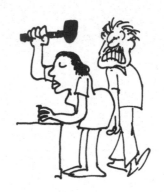

Figure 4.36. Sculptures will all have mounts made, but the exhibition will...

Figure 4.37. A padded battery housing with bolts positioning the...

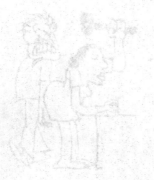

to right hand and should carry them in a wallet to keep the amount of contact to a minimum, and should also do that in no hand at all. There are a real need anyone who expects... to be just right to you. You can do a great in the... thich it carries intact straight and carry more carefully.

All figures courtesy of Amara Restoration, CPA.

SELECTED BIBLIOGRAPHY

Ahmed M, Nathi AR. IOL power determination by retinoscope. *Indian J Ophthalmol*. 1987;35(5-6):239-241.

Bigsby W, et al. Static retinoscopy results with and without a fogging lens over the non-tested eye. *Am J Optom Physiol Opt*. 1984;61(12):769-770.

Carter JH. A system of retinoscopy for the aged eye. *Am J Optom Physiol Opt*. 1986;63(4):298-299.

Duckman RH, Meyer B. Use of photoretinoscopy as a screening technique in the assessment of anisometropia and significant refractive error in infants/toddlers/children and special populations. *Am J Optom Physiol Opt*. 1987;64(8):36-49.

Gallaway M, Scheiman M. Assessment of accomodatiove facility using MEM retinoscopy. *J Am Optom Assoc*. 1990;61(8):36-39.

Hamer RD, et al. Comparison of on- and off-axis photorefraction with cycloplegic retinoscopy in infants. *J Pediatr Ophthalmol Strabismus*. 1992;29(4):232-239.

Hodi S, Wood IC. Comparison of the techniques of videorefraction and static retinoscopy in the measurement of refractive error in infants. *Ophthalmic Physiol Opt*. 1994;14(1):20-24.

Locke LC, Somers W. A comparison study of dynamic retinoscopy techniques. *Optom Vis Sci*. 1989;66(8):540-544.

Miller KM. Retinoscopy with a bent filament. *Am J Ophthalmol*. 1990;110(4):431-432.

Olver JM. Simple retinoscopic screening. *Eye*. 1988;2(pt 3):309-313.

Owens DA, et al. The effectiveness of a retinoscope beam as an accomodative stimulus. *Invest Ophthalmol Vis Sci*. 1980;19(8):942-949.

Roe LD, Guyton DL. An ophthalmoscope is not a retinoscope. The difference is in the red reflex. *Surv Ophthalmol*. 1984;28(4):345-348.

Salvesen S, Kohler M. Automated refraction. A comparative study of automated refraction with the Nidek AR-1000 autorefractor and retinoscopy. *Acta Ophthalmol (Copenh)*. 1991;69(3):342-346.

Wesson MD, et al. A comparison of cycloplegic refraction to the near retinoscopy technique for refractive error determination. *J Am Optom Assoc*. 1990;61(9):680-684.

Whitefoot H, Carman WN. Dynamic retinoscopy and accommodation. *Ophthalmic Physiol Opt*. 1992;12(1):8-17.

Wing GL. A makeshift retinoscopy rack. *Am J Ophthalmol*. 1980;89(1):142.

Zadnik K, et al. The repeatability of measurement of the ocular components. *Invest Ophthalmol Vis Sci*. 1992;33(7): 2325-2333.

SELECTED BIBLIOGRAPHY

INDEX

Printed in the United States
by Baker & Taylor Publisher Services